Differential Effects of Antidepressants

D1387545

Brian E Leonard
Department of Pharmacology
National University of Ireland, Galway
Galway, Ireland

David Healy
Department of Psychological Medicine
Hergest Unit
Ysbyty Gwynedd
Bangor, Gwynedd, UK

MARTIN DUNITZ

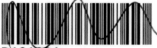

© Martin Dunitz 1999

First published in the United Kingdom
in 1999 by:

Martin Dunitz Ltd
The Livery House
7–9 Pratt Street
London NW1 0AE

A CIP record for this book is available
from the British Library.

ISBN 1-85317-657-5

Distributed in the USA, Canada and Brazil
by,

Blackwell Science Inc
Commerce Place
350 Main Street
Malden
MA02148-5018
USA
Tel: 1-800-215-1000

Printed and bound in Spain by Cayfosa.

Contents

Preface

Depression is a fairly common disorder that has a major
impact not only on the patient and society in general,
but also on the services of the general practitioner and the
psychiatrist. Partly as a result of the recent campaigns to
raise the awareness of clinicians and the general public
about the nature and extent of depression, the diagnosis
and treatment have improved. However, problems are
frequently experienced by the clinician in deciding
which, if any, of the numerous antidepressants currently
available should be used to treat a particular patient.
Questions such as the durations of treatment, the
precautions necessary when treating the elderly patient,
and which drugs are most likely to interact with the antidepressant medication also arise.

It was in an attempt to provide information in answer to
such questions that this short textbook was written. It
must be emphasized that this is not intended to be a
comprehensive overview of the subject and those inter-
ested in reading more detailed accounts are referred to
the Recommended reading list on page 99. We hope that
you, the reader, will find the contents comprehensive,

interesting and helpful to your daily clinical practice. Any comments that you may have on the contents of the text will be gratefully received.

Brian E Leonard
David Healy

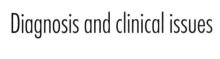

Diagnosis and clinical issues

In the mid-1950s when the antidepressants were first
discovered, there was a perception that depressive disorders were extraordinarily uncommon, of the order of
50–100 per million people; this left some of the manufacturers of the early antidepressants wondering whether
there was a market for their compounds. Now the World
Health Organization (WHO) estimates that 5–10% of the
population, that is, 100 000 000 people world wide on
any one day, may be depressed. From this increase in
the frequency of depressive disorders a number of issues
have arisen.

First, it is probably true that serious depressive disorders
or bipolar affective disorders, which require prophylactic
treatment, and severe melancholic states are only
marginally more common than they were during the
1950s. The increase in frequency in these disorders
probably owes more to increased detection rates than to
any change in methods of diagnosis or other trends.

The recognition that there were 'other' types of depression stemmed from community epidemiological work carried out in the 1960s by Michael Shepherd in the UK and subsequently by a range of epidemiological studies in the USA and Europe. These studies identified substantial psychiatric morbidity in general practice/primary care populations; this runs at an annual prevalence rate of 5–10% or more of the population or 30% of those being seen in primary care. Estimates of the lifetime prevalence of these disorders vary between 20% and 50% of the population. The precise prevalence in primary care is hard to judge because many general practitioners feel that there is a nervous component to many physical disorders – otherwise a patient would not attend the surgery. In this sense, nervousness, whether it is called anxiety or depression, leads to consultations.

For a variety of reasons, during the 1980s this nervousness, which almost certainly has a major biological component to it, came to be seen as depression rather than the 'anxiety' of the 1960s and 1970s. This probably results partly from the controversies about mass treatment of anxiety disorders with benzodiazepines. By the time the selective serotonin reuptake inhibitors (SSRIs) emerged on the market,

it would have been very difficult to call them anxiolytics. From their use in depressive disorders they became known as antidepressants, although their broad spectrum of use across, and licensed indications for use in, a range of nervous conditions from obsessive–compulsive disorder to social phobia and panic disorders, as well as depressive disorders, suggests that the SSRIs are broad-spectrum antinervous compounds.

This gives rise to a new problem: how can the action of the group of drugs originally called antidepressants be best characterized? There are several options. One is that these drugs act only as antidepressants and only work in other conditions in which there is an affective component. Another is that in the brain they have separate actions which mediate their antiobsessive, antipanic and antidepressant actions *(see Chapter 7)*. A third option, which fits the clinical observations, is that these drugs have different antinervousness actions; the antinervousness action, which is mediated by action on the serotonin (5-hydroxytryptamine or 5HT) system, is different from the action produced by drugs that are active on the noradrenergic system. The 5HT effects could be described in terms of some sort of non-sedative 'anxiolytic' action which is useful across a range of conditions, as opposed to noradrenergic effects which are more vigilant and drive enhancing.

Against this shifting background, the definitions of depression have changed. In the 1960s it was common to hear references to endogenous and reactive depressions: endogenous depressions were rare, supposedly biological in origin and only appropriately treated with pharmacotherapy; reactive or neurotic depressions were common, triggered by life events and best handled by psychotherapy. This simple picture is incorrect.

Types of depression that have biological features such as early morning wakening

and diurnal mood variation, are equally likely to be triggered by life events. Types of depression that seem to have a neurotic basis, because of an absence of biological features and a clear interplay with psychosocial difficulties, will often respond to treatment with antidepressants.

In the 1980s these shifts in understanding gave rise to the concept of major depressive disorder. The current diagnostic criteria for this are enshrined in either the Diagnostic and Statistical Manual (DSM-4) (American Psychiatric Association, 1994) or the International Classification of Diseases (ICD-10) (WHO, 1993) and are given in *Table 1*.

Table 1
Diagnostic criteria for depressive disorders in DSM-4 and ICD-10.

1 Depressed mood for most of the day
2 Markedly diminished interest in or pleasure from normal activities
3 Significant weight change — either loss or gain
4 Insomnia or hypersomnia
5 Psychomotor agitation or retardation
6 Fatigue or loss of energy
7 Feelings of worthlessness or excessive guilt
8 Reduced ability to concentrate
9 Recurrent thoughts of death or suicide

There is currently uncertainty about the interface between this condition and minor depressive disorders or chronic depressive disorders (formerly called depressive personality disorders, now termed 'dysthymia') or generalized anxiety disorder. These uncertainties in classification are somewhat academic because, in practice, all of these conditions may respond to the same range of drugs. Treatment is a balance between the risks and benefits for the individual patient.

In primary care, depressions take a number of forms. There are episodes of depression/ nervousness that appear to be reactive to life events, and treatment of these disorders with antidepressants has in general the best prognosis, because the conditions tend to be self-limiting. In such cases treatment with antidepressants is aimed at producing conditions that promote a response in those people who would normally be unlikely to respond. Angst and colleagues recently put forward this view of antidepressant actions as shown in the box.

> *The therapeutic qualities of antidepressants do not lie in the suppression of symptoms but rather are related to their ability to elicit and maintain certain conditions which allow recovery in a sub-group of patients who would otherwise remain non-responsive.*

The more severe the reaction, the more likely it is that an antidepressant will be required as *Figure 1* indicates. As illustrated, it is clear that the more severe the depressive reaction the greater the likelihood of response to treatment rather than placebo. Any active therapy involves balancing risks against benefits. The risks of treating depression involve: leaving a depressive disorder untreated; overdose from the antidepressant itself; precipitating cardiovascular or convulsive disorders; and increased nervousness leading perhaps to suicidal ideation, together with the risk of making the person worse by labelling them as depressed. The milder the depressive reaction the less likely it is that the benefits of treatment will outweigh the risk, particularly in vulnerable populations, and the greater the need for close monitoring of the patient to ensure that the hoped-for benefits have been obtained and justify the continuing risks.

In addition there is a range of other conditions, which on the one hand appear mild but, on the other are more constitutionally determined and influenced less by environmental contingencies. Some individuals are more introverted and more generally apprehensive and nervous than others, and many of these individuals end up with a diagnosis of low-grade mixed anxiety/depressive states. These people may attend the surgery frequently and

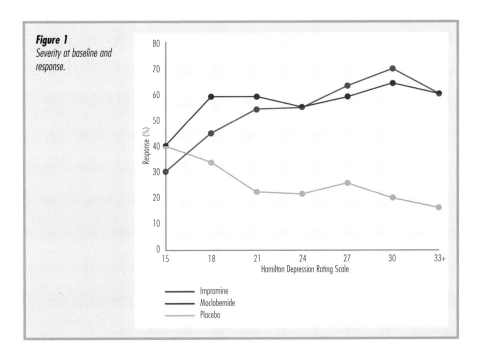

Figure 1
Severity at baseline and response.

Response (%)

Hamilton Depression Rating Scale

——— Imipramine
——— Moclobemide
·········· Placebo

attract a diagnosis of hypochondriasis or somatization disorder. A proportion of them meet the criteria for dysthymia (formerly termed 'depressive personality disorder'), whereas others will meet the criteria for social phobia. These conditions may appear mild because they have no obvious biological features; in this case drug treatment may not seem justified. However, these cases differ from milder depressive reactions in their chronicity and deserve a trial of treatment.

A significant proportion of such patients obtain modest benefits from treatment and these benefits are sustained as long as treatment is sustained. Treatment may, however, be necessary on a relatively long-term basis, unlike that in a mixed anxiety depressive reaction, where once a response has been achieved, treatment can be discontinued some time afterwards. The risks of such treatment may be consider-able, although it is now clear that patients can gain by being able to avoid alcoholism, unemployment and relationship failure, which may justify even modest improvements in overall levels of functioning.

Peter Joyce and colleagues from New Zealand carried out an intriguing set of studies which suggest that, when looking at personality-based depressions, not all antidepressants have the same effects. By comparing clomipramine with desipramine in a population of depressive individuals admitted to a district general hospital unit (with no attempt to exclude individuals on the basis of complicating personality variables), they found that personality predicted up to 50% of the variation in responsiveness to treatment. Individuals with borderline personality features responded better to clomipramine, whereas those with asthenic or dependent personality features responded better to desipramine. The responsiveness of forms of social phobia to monoamine oxidase inhibitors (MAOIs) and SSRIs is also of interest here. Clinical trials with these drugs have indicated that those individuals with severe forms of social phobia that merge into avoidant personality disorder often do as well as those with the milder forms. These results underpin hitherto unspecified clinical impressions that, for some, MAOIs may have personality-strengthening properties.

The therapeutic question

Given the relative safety of most modern antidepressants and the difficulties in clearly delineating types of nervousness that will respond specifically to individual drugs, what principles should guide therapy? A number can be offered. In those with a mild condition, there are risks in making a formal diagnosis, particularly in a referral to a mental health team. Unless they lead on to interventions that produce clear benefits, diagnoses can compromise future career and relationship prospects. Treatment of the condition with pharmacotherapy, but diagnosing a condition as a stress-related disorder may avoid some of these difficulties. Management by a counsellor in a primary care setting may also achieve the same end, although management by a counsellor in a mental health team setting can offer all the stigma of a mental illness diagnosis with none of the benefits of an effective intervention.

On initiation of treatment, certain principles should guide it. Although relatively safe, antidepressant treatments are not innocuous. A clearcut therapeutic response justifies continuing with treatment, but what happens if there is no clear response? From the outset, it is appropriate to indicate to the patient what the treatment goals are: reduction of anxiety levels, improvement of sleep, restoration of energy, etc. It is also appropriate to indicate the length of the treatment and what can be done if there is no response in this time. These principles should apply regardless of the therapeutic modality — pharmacotherapy or psychotherapy/counselling.

If the patient fails to comply, this could be the result of several things: treatment-induced side-effects; clash between the patient's and the physician's explanatory models; or a rejection of the physician's style. It is therefore, very important, to establish how the patient views his or her problem and, where possible, to accommodate any therapy within that framework.

Assessing clinical outcomes

2

In a recent clinical trial comparing reboxetine, fluoxetine and placebo, using conventional measures of antidepressant efficacy such as the Hamilton Rating Scale for Depression (HAM-D) and a Social Adaptation Self Evaluation Scale (SASS), results for the two drugs were the same. But there were clear differences between reboxetine and fluoxetine at the end of the trial period on the SASS *(see Figure 2)*. This result is of more than usual significance to primary care physicians and clinical psychiatrists for a number of reasons. First, it is not readily compatible with simplistic notions of a monoamine 'lesion' in depressive disorders. Second, it suggests that there may be differences in the profile of patients who benefit from one particular group of antidepressants. Third, the result suggests that there may be differences between antidepressants in the quality of life they deliver to patients in ways that have practical implications.

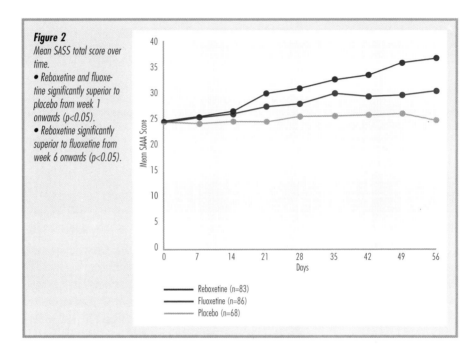

Figure 2
Mean SASS total score over time.
• Reboxetine and fluoxetine significantly superior to placebo from week 1 onwards (p<0.05).
• Reboxetine significantly superior to fluoxetine from week 6 onwards (p<0.05).

Reboxetine (n=83)
Fluoxetine (n=86)
Placebo (n=68)

There are five ways to assess whether an antidepressant is working:

1. Through use of observer-based disease-specific rating scales, e.g. the HAM-D *(Table 2)*.

2. Through use of patient-based disease-specific rating scales, e.g. the Beck Depression Inventory (BDI) *(Table 3)*.

3. Through use of observer-based scales that are not specific to any one disease. This format underpins the Clinical Global Impression scales and the observer-based Social Adaptation Scale *(Table 4)*.

4. Through use of what are in essence patient-based global impression scales, e.g. the SASS. This group also includes

Table 2
Observer rating scales: disease specific.

- Hamilton Rating Scale for Depression (HAM-D)
- Montgomery–Asberg Depression Rating Scale
- Clinical Interview for Depression
- Beck Depression Scale
- Raskin Severity of Depression Scale
- Inventory of Depressive Symptomatology

Table 3
Subjective rating scales: disease specific.

- Beck Depression Inventory (BDI)
- Zung Self-rated Depression Scale
- Inventory of Depressive Symptomatology

Table 4
Observer rating scales: disease non-specific

- Clinical Global Impression
- Clinical Global Improvement Scale
- Clinical Global Assessment of Functioning
- Social Adaptation Scale

explicit and implicit quality of life measures *(Tables 5 and 6)*.

5. Outcome measures such as suicide rates *(see Chapter 11)*.

Observer-based disease-specific rating scales function like the column of mercury in a syphgmomanometer. Unless the figures on these scales fall, the drug in question is not an antidepressant. Just as a reduction in blood pressure reading can be achieved in a variety of ways using anti-hypertensives, and different treatments can produce a variety of longer-term outcomes and differential quality of life outcomes, so antidepressants should be considered as a heterogeneous class of agents that achieve their benefits in various distinctive ways.

Table 5
Self-rating scales: disease non-specific.

- Psychological Well-being Scale
- PCASEE
- SF-36
- Quality of Life in Depression Scale
- Sertraline Quality of Life Battery
- Quality of Life, Enjoyment and Satisfaction
- Social Adaptation Self Evaluation Scale (SASS)

Table 6
The SASS and the HAM-D.

	SASS	HAM-D
Completed by patient	+	0
Completed by doctor	0	+
Measures symptoms	0	+
Measures daily activities	+	0
Usable in GP clinic	+	0

The impression that all antidepressants are the same – indistinguishable except for their side-effects – probably stemmed from the fact that, on scales such as the HAM-D, they produce similar drops in depression scores in mild-to-moderate cases of depression. However, before the widespread introduction of the HAM-D, clinical global impressions in the 1960s were that these agents were not the same and indeed these perceptions of difference underpinned the development of the SSRIs.

There is some evidence from clinical trials that when patient-based measures, such as the BDI, are used depressed patients prefer the outcomes produced by drugs selective to noradrenergic systems rather than those that are selective to serotonergic systems. This makes a certain amount of sense because clinical impression is that types of depression not dominated by anxiety show a quicker response to those antidepressants that have a noradrenergic component; these types of depression are the ones most likely to be recruited into clinical trials. There have been no such studies in anxiety states, but they could well produce quite different results.

Against this background, the results obtained for reboxetine and fluoxetine with the SASS are significant. Quality of life was introduced as a concept into medicine in the mid-1960s for patients who underwent renal dialysis; it was recognized that a treatment could be life-saving and yet produce an outcome that left a lot to be desired. The concept was developed further in areas such as anti-hypertensive therapy. A study by Jachuk in 1982 indicated that, although a treatment might lower the 'mercury column', that is, the observer-based rating, the patient or relative might see a different set of outcomes. Patient-based assessments revealed that someone could become hypochondriacal and develop symptoms not previously present, just as a result of the side-effects. In the case of hypertension the angiotensin-converting enzyme

(ACE) inhibitors subsequently found a market because of the better quality of life they produced.

What might be revealed by the SASS finding?

Since the development of observer-based social function scales, it has been claimed that antidepressant therapy is able to correct the core features of depressive disorders within 2–3 weeks, but it takes several weeks or even months for social function to return to normal. From the SASS, there is a suggestion that reboxetine produces a much more rapid return to normal, but it remains to be seen whether this is confirmed by observer-based measures.

Social functioning and quality of life are also related to the burden of the side-effects of the treatment. Currently, the true frequency, intensity or full range of side-effects of any psychotropic agent is not known, because the reporting of side-effects in clinical trials has been dependent on the collection of spontaneous reports from patients. We see an example of this in the reports of sexual dysfunction in patients taking SSRIs; in the original reports sexual dysfunction was about 5%, but in subsequent systematic investigations, the estimates rose to 50%. A number of companies have started to incorporate systematic ratings of side-effects in all their trials, using scales such as the UKU (a monitoring scale for side-effects developed by the Scandinavian Society for Psychopharmacology). Until data are available from these studies, findings on scales such as the SASS and quality of life (QoL) instruments offer probably the best estimate of the full impact of drug treatment on patients.

The burden of side-effects is reflected in an instrument such as the SASS, but there are probably other factors at play. Agents active on noradrenergic systems are more likely to enhance vigilance and restore energy than agents active on serotonin (5-hydroxytryptamine or 5HT) systems and, for this reason, the effects of an agent such as reboxetine may produce a better quality of life for some patients than the 'sanguinity-inducing' effects of the SSRIs. An experiment might bring this home. In the case of obsessive–compulsive disorder, for instance, patients report that one of the beneficial effects of SSRIs is that these agents take the edge off intrusive thoughts, so that they recede into the background or

disappear completely. There is evidence that these drugs have such effects even in healthy volunteers. Based on this, social functioning, which depends partly on an appropriate level of concern about relationships, careers, overdrafts and other challenges/problems, could therefore be adversely affected by an SSRI. Consistent with these findings from healthy volunteers, there have been indications for some time that a proportion of those whose core symptoms clear up on SSRIs but who do not rate themselves as back to normal have a certain amount of 'emotional blunting'. This has been, to date, a relatively unexplored side-effect of SSRIs.

It is noteworthy that the development of QoL scales in the early 1990s was sponsored by many of the manufacturers of SSRIs. This sponsorship was based on the reasonable expectation that, although the SSRIs might have no better treatment effects than the older tricyclic antidepressants (TCAs), they would result in a better quality of life by triggering off fewer side-effects. This assumption that there are fewer side-effects after treatment with SSRIs, compared with TCAs, is a notional rather than a proven one. It was underpinned by the idea that TCAs acted on many different systems, many of which were not essential for the therapeutic effects of the drug, whereas the SSRIs acted on fewer systems, so there would be fewer side-effects. This overlooks the fact that side-effects can arise through drug action on the primary system, with more potent actions on this system leading to more devastating side-effects. In the case of the SSRIs, these side-effects include nausea sufficiently severe to stop treatment, sexual dysfunction which arises in 50% of those on the treatment, or akathisia and dyskinesias both of which can lead to secondary complications. The results on quality of life instruments for SSRIs have in general been disappointing, which supports the previous point. They are in line with the findings for fluoxetine on the SASS: treatment may produce some benefits but it does not appear to restore all responders to normal. Care must be taken in interpreting average figures on quality of life and SASS instruments, as there are two possible interpretations. One is that all patients do slightly better on noradrenergic agents, and the other is that a larger proportion of patients may, for example, do better on reboxetine, although a significant proportion of patients may also recover fully on fluoxetine. Currently, the data suggests that the latter interpretation is closer to the mark.

What are the implications for clinical practice?

As a consequence of both the educational campaigns to detect and diagnose depression and the observer-based scales, which have focused heavily on the core features of the illness (sleep, appetite and energy disturbances, as well as guilt and suicidal thoughts), clinicians in both primary care and hospital practice have probably been guilty of checking these core features only when patients return for an assessment. When they find that these features are improved, they have assumed that the patient is well and have advised them to continue treatment for anything from 3 to 12 months. There would seem to be a place here for not just assessing whether the patient is well, but for trying to determine whether he or she is now 'normal'.

Some individuals indicate that there have been substantial improvements, but they are not normal, either because they feel too detached or apathetic or because of a variety of other reasons such as feeling unreal. Such factors probably play a part in those patients who stop treatment, even though they have a good relationship with their clinician and do not have any obvious side-effects such as nausea, dry mouth or urinary retention. The danger in this, with any antidepressant, but particularly with an SSRI, is that the patient may then experience discontinuation effects that could have been managed far better if discontinuation had been planned.

When assessing the evidence from clinical trials, what emerges is not necessarily evidence-based practice, at least in psychiatry. The subjects recruited for depression studies are termed 'subjects of convenience'; they are not usually on any other treatment, they are not ill in any other way and they have no significant personality disturbances. In practice the individuals being treated in primary care may have multiple problems, difficult psychosocial situations and treatment may be complicated by a range of medications being taken concurrently, if only the oral contraceptive pill or hormone replacement therapy (HRT). There is very little medicine-based evidence and against this background treatments that show evidence of efficacy on a range of measures from observer-based disease-specific scales to quality of life instruments can be recommended, but there is still a place for clinical impressions. It is only when a drug is available for use that proper clinical impressions can be drawn. It should also be remembered that an astutely observed side-effect can provide the basis for future therapies.

Against this background of evidence, a lot of which has little basis in typical clinical practice, 'hard outcome' measures such as suicide or deaths on antidepressants have considerable importance. A good example is given by studies of some of the early lipid-lowering agents: some of these clearly lowered lipid levels in the short term but did not prolong life in the longer term. The studies on suicide discussed in *Chapter 11* offer some encouragement for the use of noradrenergic-selective agents; however, constant vigilance, particularly in the first few weeks of treatment, is called for when delivering any treatment including psychotherapy.

Basic concepts of neurotransmission in the brain

3

It has been accepted for about 100 years that communication between neurons in the brain is primarily chemical. In recent years, it has become established that over 50 neurotransmitters and neuromodulators are present in the mammalian brain, all of which fulfil different physiological functions. The neurotransmitters can be broadly divided into the 'classic' neurotransmitters such as acetylcholine, noradrenaline, dopamine, serotonin (5-hydroxytryptamine), γ-aminobutyric acid (GABA), glutamic acid, aspartic acid, histamine and adrenaline, and the numerous neuropeptides (such as enkephalin, endorphins, corticotrophin-releasing factor (CRF), tachykines) and trace amines (such as tryptamine and phenylethylamine), which also play a role in central neurotransmission. *Table 7* summarizes the main neurotransmitters found in the brain.

It is well established that these neurotranmitters have specific physiological functions which are dictated by the neuronal networks that they excite or inhibit within

Table 7
Principal neurotransmitters and neuromodulators found in the human brain.

Amines	Opioid peptides
Serotonin (5-hydroxytryptamine, 5HT)	Met-enkephalin
Noradrenaline (NA)	Leu-enkephalin
Dopamine (DA)	Dynorphin
Adrenaline (A)	β-Endorphin
Choline ester	**Gastrointestinal hormones in brain**
Acetylcholine (Ach)	Cholecystokinin (CCK)
Amino acids	Gastrin
	Secretion
γ-Aminobutyric acid (GABA)	Substance P
Glutamic acid	Vasoactive intestinal peptide (VIP)
Aspartic acid	
Glycine	**Others**
	Neuropeptide Y (NPY)
Pituitary peptides	Neurotensin
	Prolactin
Corticotrophin (ACTH)	Prostaglandins
Growth hormone (GH)	
α-Melanocyte-stimulating hormone (α-MSH)	
Oxytocin	*This list is incomplete. Over 50 different*
Vasopressin	*neuroactive molecules have already been*
Corticotrophin-releasing factor (CRF)	*identified. The amines, acetylcholine and the*
Somatostatin	*amino acid neurotransmitters are some-*
Thyrotrophin-releasing hormone (TRH)	*times termed 'classic' transmitters.*

the brain. Whether a particular neuronal pathway is excited or inhibited depends on the nature of the receptor upon which the transmitter acts. In brief, neurotrans- mitters can excite or inhibit nerve cells. Thus, transmitters such as glutamate can cause excitation by activating one of the many glutamergic receptors that are widely distributed throughout the brain. These fall into two major categories and it depends upon the nature of the specific receptor whether a fast response (micro to milliseconds) or a slow response (milliseconds to seconds) occurs. For example, the N-methyl-D-asparate (NMDA) receptor is linked directly to an ion channel in the nerve membrane. On stimulating the NMDA receptor, the ion channel opens causing a rapid membrane depolarization. This then causes a wave of excitation to move down the axon, resulting in the enhanced release of the neurotransmitter for the nerve terminal. By contrast, stimulation of the glutamergic metabotropic receptors leads to a much slower excitatory response because the change in neuronal activity depends upon the stimulation of second messengers within the nerve cell. Thus a slower excitatory response occurs. These different mechanisms that govern 'fast' and 'slow' transmitted responses are illustrated diagrammatically in *Figures 3 and 4*.

In addition to the 'fast' transmitters, which are excitatory in their action depending upon the nature of the receptor on which they act, inhibitory transmitters also have an important function in the brain. The amino acids GABA and glycine are exam-ples of inhibitory transmitters in several regions of the brain. Inhibitory receptors may also be ionotropic or metabotropic in nature (that is, 'fast' or 'slow'). GABA produces a 'fast' inhibitory response by hyperpolarizing the nerve cell. This means that instead of Na^+ and K^+ ions being exchanged across the nerve membrane as happens after the activation of an excitatory receptor, K^+ and Cl^- ions enter the cell after GABA activates the ionotropic GABA-A receptor, thereby hyperpolarizing the cell and reducing neuronal function. A list of the main excitatory and inhibitory receptors is shown in *Table 8*.

In addition to the excitatory and inhibitory neurotransmitters, several neuromodulators are also present in the mammalian brain; their functions appear to be to enhance or reduce the physiological response caused by a conventional transmitter. For example, in the basal ganglia, dopamine coexists with the peptide cholecystokinin (CCK). When CCK is co-released with dopamine, the physiological response of the dopamine receptor is enhanced. This finding led to the hypothesis that CCK receptor antagonists may reduce the functional activity of the dopaminergic system and therefore have some therapeutic value in the treatment of schizo-

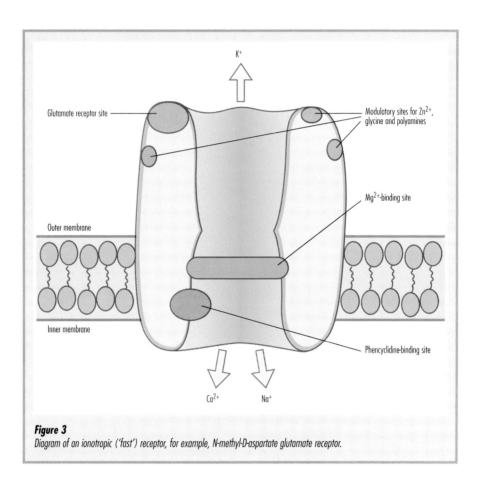

Figure 3
Diagram of an ionotropic ('fast') receptor, for example, N-methyl-D-aspartate glutamate receptor.

phrenia, in which dopaminergic function may be enhanced.

The link between the various neurotransmitter systems in the brain is an important mechanism by which one transmitter system may increase or decrease the functional activity of another system with which it is in contact. This can be achieved by the presence of heteroceptors located on nerve terminals. An example of such a link between the adrenergic and seroton-

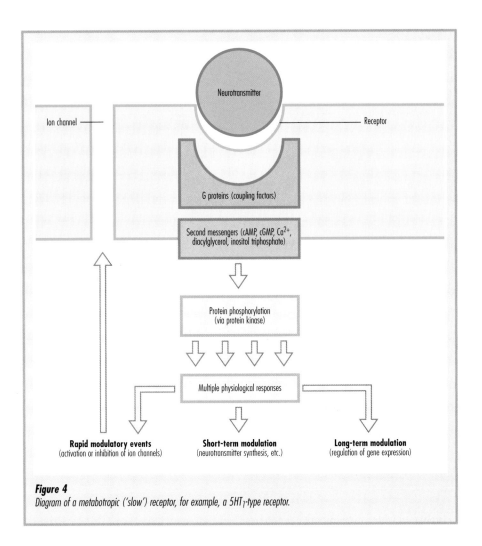

Figure 4
Diagram of a metabotropic ('slow') receptor, for example, a 5HT₁-type receptor.

Table 8
Some of the main excitatory and inhibitory receptors in the human brain.

1   Fast ion-channel linked receptors (ionotropic receptors)
    Cholinergic nicotinic receptors[a]
    γ-Amino butyrate (GABA) type A receptors[b]
    Glutamate/aspartate (NMDA type) receptors[b]
    $5HT_3$-receptors
2   Slow receptors linked to G proteins (metabotropic receptors)
    Cholinergic muscarinic receptors
    Adrenergic:
        α_1-receptors[b]
        α_2-receptors[b]
        β_1-receptors[a]
        β_2-receptors[a]
    Dopamine (D_1, D_2, D_3, D_4, D_5) receptors
    GABA type B receptors
    Glutamate (metabotropic receptors)
    Histamine type 1, 2, 3 receptors
    Serotonin: $5HT_1$, $5HT_2$, $5HT_3$, $5HT_4$, $5HT_5$, $5HT_6$, $5HT_7$.
    Peptide receptors: angiotensin II, cholecystokinin A and B, vasopressin, opioids.

[a] *Mainly excitatory receptors.*
[b] *Mainly inhibitory receptors.*
The physiological response elicited by the other receptors may be excitatory or inhibitory, depending on their location and function in the brain. For example, $5HT_{1A}$-receptors on the nerve cell are inhibitory whereas the postsynaptic $5HT_{1A}$-receptors are mainly excitatory.

ergic system in the brain is illustrated diagrammatically in *Figure 5*. Noradrenaline is shown to activate the α_2-heteroceptors located in a serotonergic nerve terminal. As a result, the release of serotonin is decreased, suggesting that the α_2-heteroceptor has an inhibitory action on the release of serotonin. The novel

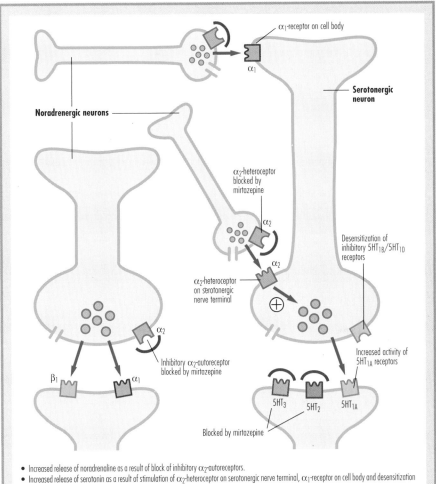

- Increased release of noradrenaline as a result of block of inhibitory α_2-autoreceptors.
- Increased release of serotonin as a result of stimulation of α_2-heteroceptor on serotonergic nerve terminal, α_1-receptor on cell body and desensitization of inhibitory $5HT_{1B}/5HT_{1D}$ receptor on serotonergic terminal.
- Net effect: enhanced noradrenergic and serotonergic.

Figure 5
'Cross-talk' between the noradrenergic and serotonergic system and how it helps to explain the mode of action of the tetracyclic antidepressant mirtazepine.

tetracyclic antidepressant mirtazapine acts as an antagonist at noradrenergic and serotonergic receptors. By blocking the inhibitory α_2-adrenoceptors on both noradrenergic and serotonergic terminals, mirtazapine enhances the release of noradrenaline from noradrenergic and serotonergic terminals. This example illustrates the importance of 'cross-talk' between different neurotransmitter systems and shows how it can be used in the development of new therapeutic strategies for the treatment of depression.

Summary

Neurotransmitters in the mammalian brain may be divided into the 'classic' neurotransmitters, such as acetylcholine, noradrenaline, serotonin, dopamine, glutamate and GABA, and the neuromodulators and trace transmitters, which include such peptides as the enkephalins and tryptamine. These neurotransmitters and neuromodulators elicit their physiological responses by acting on specific receptors. Whether the response is fast (microseconds) or slow (milliseconds) depends on the nature of the receptor upon which they act. Fast receptors are known as ionotropic receptors and their direct activation leads to the opening of the ion channel in the nerve membrane. Slow receptors are known as metabotropic receptors and their activation initiates changes within the nerve cell whereby second messengers (for example cyclic AMP) are produced. These highly reactive molecules phosphorylate membrane proteins to open the ion channel. In addition to the fast and slow transmitters and their receptors, neuromodulators act either to enhance or to reduce the action of classic transmitters on their receptors. Cross-talk between different neurotransmitter systems can occur where one transmitter activates a heteroceptor located on the terminal of another transmitter system. This may lead to an increase or decrease in the release of the second transmitter, depending on the nature of the heteroceptor.

Biochemical basis of depression

4

The amine hypothesis

For over 30 years it has been widely accepted that the symptoms of depression arise as a consequence of a disturbance of one or more of the biogenic amine neurotransmitters in the brain. This forms the basis of the monoamine hypothesis of depression, which suggests that a relative deficit in noradrenaline, serotonin and possibly dopamine in the limbic (emotional) regions of the brain is primarily responsible for the symptoms of depression.

Despite the popularity of the monoamine hypothesis, direct evidence for a primary deficit in such neurotransmitters in depression is limited. Nevertheless, there is some evidence, for this deficit, from the postmortem studies on the brains of patients who committed suicide, from cerebrospinal fluid analyses of depressed patients, from endocrine studies in which the pituitary–adrenal axis responds subnormally to a challenge with specific noradrenergic or serotonergic drugs such as clonidine or fenfluramine and, lastly, from changes in noradrenaline and serotonin receptor function on platelet and lymphocyte membranes in depressed patients. More recently, positron emission tomography (PET) studies have shown direct evidence that a subpopulation of serotonin receptors ($5HT_{2A}$) is present at a higher density in the limbic region of the brain of the depressed patient.

Summary

The monoamine hypothesis of depression postulates that the changes in mood (possibly linked to a defect in serotonin and dopamine), drive and motivation (possibly noradrenaline and dopamine linked) are the result of a hypoactivity of the main monoamine neurotransmitters in the emotional areas of the brain.

It must be stressed, however, that this is a gross oversimplification of the situation, because it has been shown that many other neurotransmitters are changed in the brains of depressed patients, in addition to the three monoamines that have received most attention.

Antidepressant drugs and the amine hypothesis

Support for the monoamine hypothesis initially arose over 30 years ago with the accidental finding that the antihypertensive drug reserpine (from the root of the Indian snake plant *Rauwolfia serpentia*) lowered the blood pressure but also, in some patients, caused sedation and a depressed mood. Subsequently, it was found that reserpine depleted the central and peripheral nerve terminals of noradrenaline, serotonin and depramine. At about this time, the first two effective antidepressants to be discovered (the tricyclic antidepressant imipramine and the monoamine oxidase inhibitor iproniazid) were shown to enhance the activity of noradrenaline and serotonin in the brain. Other psychotropic drugs such as the stimulant amphetamines and cocaine were shown to cause euphoria and excitement by specifically releasing noradrenaline and dopamine (amphetamine) or inhibiting the reuptake of these amines (cocaine) in the limbic regions of the brain. However, such drugs, unlike the antidepressants, only produced temporary relief of the depressed mood because, by their action, they reduced the amine content of the nerve terminals. Thus effective antidepressants were shown to alter the kinetics of the monoamines so that their physiological actions could be sustained and in this way lead to a normalization of the mood state.

Antidepressants act on various biochemical processes in the brain by which the amine neurotransmitters prolong their physiological actions and thereby attenuate the main symptoms of depression.

How do antidepressants improve amine function?

Soon after the discovery of the therapeutic efficacy of imipramine and iproniazid, it was shown from studies in experimental animals that these drugs acted in different ways on the monoamine nerve terminals to preserve their duration of action. For over 60 years it had been known that the enzyme monoamine oxidase catalysed the breakdown of monoamines (such as noradrenaline, serotonin, dopamine) and the 'trace' amines (for example, tyramine and tryptamine) that are present in the diet and in minute quantities in the brain. It was subsequently shown that monoamine oxidase occurred in nerve terminals as well as in the liver, platelets, the gastrointestinal tract and elsewhere in the body. Thus by inhibiting the activity of this enzyme irreversibly, iproniazid could largely prevent the breakdown of the endogenous amine transmitters. This led to an accumulation of the amines in the nerve terminals, so that an increased quantity of the transmitter would be released after the passage of the nerve impulse. This provided a simplified explanation of how monoamine oxidase inhibitors (MAOIs) probably reversed many of the main symptoms of depression.

Imipramine was the first major therapeutic advance in the treatment of depression and its possible mode of action was indicated by its ability to enhance the hypertensive effect of noradrenaline on the blood pressure of the cat. It was subsequently shown that imipramine potentiated the action of noradrenaline by inhibiting the reuptake of the amine into the sympathetic nerve terminal; in this way it prolonged the action of the amine on the vasoconstrictor α_1-adrenoceptors of the blood vessels. Further experimental studies showed that imipramine, and all the closely related TCAs, impeded the reuptake of noradrenaline and serotonin into neurons for the brain. It was also shown that some TCAs were more effective in inhibiting noradrenaline (for example, desipramine, nortriptyline) than serotonin whereas others preferentially inhibited serotonin reuptake (for example, clomipramine).

More recently, antidepressants have been developed that show a high degree of selectivity in inhibiting noradrenaline reuptake (such as reboxetine) or serotonin (as exemplified by fluoxetine and the other SSRIs).

In addition, to avoid the numerous adverse effects of the TCAs, antidepressants have been developed that are potent inhibitors of both noradrenaline and serotonin, but which do not affect the muscarinic, α_1-adrenergic or H_1-receptors. These include venlafaxin and milnacipran.

The tetracyclic antidepressant, mianserin, was discovered some 30 years ago which lacked MAO inhibitory properties and did not have any significant effect on amine reuptake. Mianserin was subsequently shown to block the inhibitory presynaptic α_2-adrenoceptor and also the postsynaptic $5HT_{2A}$-receptor. The possible importance of this action is discussed later, but suffice it to say that such an action results in a facilitation of both central noradrenergic and serotonergic function. A more potent analogue of mianserin, mirtazapine, has recently been marketed. This has an improved side-effect profile over mianserin but its mechanism of action is essentially similar to the older drug.

There are a number of novel antidepressants that act as partial agonists on $5HT_{1A}$-receptors in the higher centres of the brain. These include ipsapirone and flesinoxan. The mechanism of action of these drugs has been described in terms of their ability to desensitize the inhibitory $5HT_{1A}$-receptors on the serotonergic cell bodies. This action results in a facilitation of serotonin release from the nerve terminals in the frontal cortex.

In addition to the SSRIs that inhibit serotonin reuptake, tianeptine has recently been marketed in France. So far this is a unique antidepressant in that initially it enhances the reuptake of serotonin into central neurons, but after chronic administration it appears to facilitate serotonergic neurotransmission.

Summary

After their acute administration, different classes of antidepressant have been shown to facilitate central noradrenergic or serotonergic transmission by inhibiting amine catabolism (MAOIs) and inhibiting amine reuptake thereby prolonging the actions of the amines at postsynaptic receptor sites (TCAs, SSRIs, venlafazine; reboxetine, etc), or by selectively enhancing noradrenaline release and modulating serotonin action postsynaptically (for example, mianserin and mirtazapine).

Why is there a delay between the start of antidepressant treatment and the onset of the therapeutic effect?

It soon became apparent, after the introduction of the first effective antidepressants some 40 years ago, that there is generally a delay of 2–3 weeks before they become optimally effective. At first it was thought that the delay in onset was the result of the time it takes for the drug to get into the brain to produce changes in the central neurotransmitters. However, pharmacokinetic studies suggest that this is an unlikely explanation. Furthermore, the effects of the antidepressants on the reuptake processes, amine release mechanism or MAO are rapid, so it must be concluded that these acute effects are necessary but not in themselves an explanation. The most plausible reason for the delay in onset relates to the changes in pre- and postsynaptic receptor function which occur as a consequence of the alteration in monoamine dynamics which follows the chronic administration of the

antidepressant. For example, some 20 years ago it was shown that the density of β-adrenoceptors in the frontal cortex decreases after chronic administration of most types of antidepressants. This change approximately paralleled the time taken for the therapeutic effect to become manifest. Subsequently, it was shown that other neurotransmitter receptors also change in response to chronic antidepressant treatment. Thus, $5HT_{1A}$, $5HT_{2A}$, N-methyl-D-aspartate (NMDA) glutamate receptors, γ-aminobutyrate type B receptors and various neuropeptide receptors have also been shown to change their density and functional activity at a time that approximates the onset of therapeutic effect.

The monoamine hypothesis of depression has therefore been modified to become the receptor sensitivity hypothesis, to reflect the adaptive changes in different neurotransmitter receptors which occur in response to the altered monoamine dynamics after the reduction in amine reuptake. This is discussed later.

Summary

The delay in the onset of the therapeutic response to an antidepressant appears to coincide with changes in different types of neurotransmitter receptors which may be functionally abnormal in the brain of the depressed patient. Even though the antidepressant may show selectivity for one particular neurotransmitter system (for example, serotonin in the case of the SSRIs or noradrenaline after reboxetine administration), there is evidence that other receptors also change in addition to those occupied by serotonin or noradrenaline. This suggests that many different neurotransmitters interact in the brain and that the depressed patient shows a response to antidepressant treatment only when these systems start to normalize.

Treatment of depression and the quality of life of the patient

It is now well established that a patient with major depression often has physical ill-health. One of the causes of this relates to the coincidental suppression of immune function which renders the patient liable to infections and at an increased risk of cancer. Anecdotal reports of a higher incidence of death from various forms of cancer have appeared in the literature for the past 2000 years. It is now known that the body's defence against infections and cancer is largely the result of different types of T-cells. T-cell function, and anti-body production, are reduced in the untreated depressed patient. Although this may result partly from the hypersecretion of cortisol, which characterizes the depressed patient, it is now established that there is increased secretion of various cytokines in the depressed patient. These cytokines not only affect the peripheral immune system but can also act as immunotransmitters in the brain. In this way the cytokines can enhance corticotrophin-releasing factor (CRF) release and prostaglandin synthesis. The prostaglandins are known to reduce the release of brain monoamines thereby further enhancing the neurotransmitter deficit that underlies the depressed state. After effective treatment of the depressed patient, the immune system largely returns to normal.

The interrelationship of the immune, endocrine and neurotransmitter behaviours forms the basis of psychoneuroimmunology and raises the idea of depression being a 'whole body' disease. Effective treatment of depression with antidepressants thus not only improves the mood of the patient, but also contributes indirectly to the improved quality of life. The possible relationship between the biochemical changes in depression and the mode of action of antidepressants is shown in *Figure 6*.

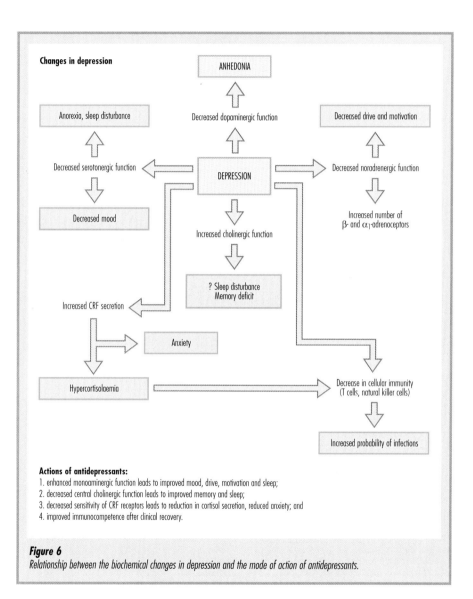

Figure 6
Relationship between the biochemical changes in depression and the mode of action of antidepressants.

Pharmacological properties and side-effects of antidepressants: an overview

5

The development of effective antidepressants in the 1950s, which were subsequently found to inhibit the reuptake of noradrenaline and serotonin into the nerve terminal, helped to lay the foundation of the monoamine theory of depression. Evidence has already been presented implicating changes in both noradrenergic and serotonergic function in the untreated depressed patient. Antidepressants may therefore be classified in terms of their chemical structure or acute effects on amine neurotransmitters. It would be anticipated that there is a correlation between the structure of an antidepressant and its biological actions. However, so far there is no evidence to support such a view so that evidence for antidepressant efficacy is largely dependent on the outcome of clinical studies. It should perhaps be added that some rodent models which are based on chronic antidepressant-induced changes in behaviour after specific lesions to the limbic system, have been shown to have predictive validity for the detection of new antidepressants.

The historical development of the antidepressant is summarized in *Table 9*. Their therapeutic actions are usually explained by the mechanism by which they enhance monoamine function in the brain. Thus, most of the TCAs and the serotonin and noradrenaline reuptake inhibitors (SNRIs), such as venlafaxine and milnacipran, inhibit both noradrenaline and serotonin reuptake. Conversely, the SSRIs, such as fluoxetine, and the noradrenaline reuptake inhibitors (NARIs), as exemplified by reboxetine, show selectivity in inhibiting serotonin and noradrenaline respectively. Monoamine oxidase inhibitors (MAOIs), at therapeutically effective doses, inhibit the metabolism of noradrenaline and serotonin, whereas the tetracyclic antidepressants mianserin and mirtazapine have little effect on the amine reuptake sites, but enhance the release of noradrenaline and facilitate serotonergic function indirectly by blocking the inhibitory α_2-adrenergic autoreceptors and stimulating the postsynaptic 5-hydroxytryptamine $5HT_{1A}$-receptors. Several second-generation antidepressants have actions that prevent their classification into these well-defined groups. Trazodone, for example, is a weak inhibitor of serotonin reuptake and can increase noradrenaline release as a result of its antagonistic action on presynaptic α_2-adrenoceptors. It also blocks postsynaptic $5HT_2$-receptors, an action shared with mianserin and mirtazapine.

Unlike noradrenaline and serotonin, much less attention has been given to the action of antidepressants on dopaminergic function. Of the antidepressants available

1957–70	TCAs	Tricyclic antidepressants
	MAOIs	Non-selective monoamine oxidase inhibitors
1970–80	NARIs	Noradrenaline reuptake inhibitors
1980–90	SSRIs	Selective serotonin reuptake inhibitors
1990–2000	RIMAs	Reversible inhibitors of monoamine oxidase
	SNRIs	Serotonin and noradrenaline reuptake
	NASSAs	Noradrenergic and specific serotonergic antidepressants
	Selective NARIs	Selective noradrenaline reuptake inhibitors

Table 9
Antidepressants and acronyms.

in Europe, only nomifensin was shown to enhance brain noradrenergic and dopaminergic function by inhibiting the reuptake of these transmitters. However, nomifensin was withdrawn because of the rare occurrence of haemolytic anaemia. Buproprion is available in the USA and has been shown to enhance dopaminergic function by inhibiting the transmitter reuptake. Amoxepine also has some dopamine uptake inhibitory action but, being structurally related to the neuroleptic loxepine, it has also been shown to block postsynaptic dopamine receptors and cause extrapyramidal side-effects. It could be anticipated that drugs which facilitate dopaminergic function would also cause hyperactivity, euphoria and excitement and therefore have limited value in the treatment of depression. Cocaine and the stimulating amphetamines are examples of drugs that potentiate dopaminergic function and are well established as drugs of abuse. The actions of the different classes of antidepressants on monoamine function in the brain are summarized in **Figures 7–12**.

Side-effects of antidepressants

The principal difference between the first – and second – generation antidepressants

relates to the frequency and severity of their side-effects. Most of these side-effects are explicable, in terms of their direct action on serotonergic and noradrenergic receptors.

Tricyclic antidepressants (TCAs)

* Consequences of blockade of muscarinic receptors (atropine-like effect): dry mouth, blurred vision, raised intraocular pressure, urinary retention, constipation, tachycardia, confusion.

* Consequence of blockade of α_1-adrenoceptors: orthostatic hypotension, dizziness.

* Consequence of blockade of H_1-receptor: sedation, ? weight gain.

* Other effects include reduced sexual function. However, cardiotoxicity, particularly in elderly patients and if taken in overdose, arises from cardiac conduction block (quinidine-like effect).

Profuse sweating is also a major problem with the TCAs. When they are withdrawn abruptly, there is evidence of increased gastrointestinal activity (diarrhoea, nausea, etc.). These side-effects of the TCAs are directly related to their action on muscarinic (mainly M_1), histamine (H_1) and adrenergic (α_1) receptors.

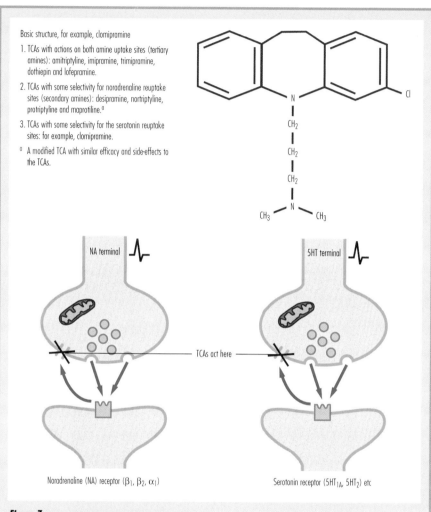

Basic structure, for example, clomipramine

1. TCAs with actions on both amine uptake sites (tertiary amines): amitriptyline, imipramine, trimipramine, dothiepin and lofepramine.

2. TCAs with some selectivity for noradrenaline reuptake sites (secondary amines): desipramine, nortriptyline, protriptyline and maprotiline.[a]

3. TCAs with some selectivity for the serotonin reuptake sites: for example, clomipramine.

[a] A modified TCA with similar efficacy and side-effects to the TCAs.

NA terminal

5HT terminal

TCAs act here

Noradrenaline (NA) receptor (β_1, β_2, α_1)

Serotonin receptor ($5HT_{1A}$, $5HT_2$) etc

Figure 7
Action of tricyclic antidepressants on monoamine reuptake.

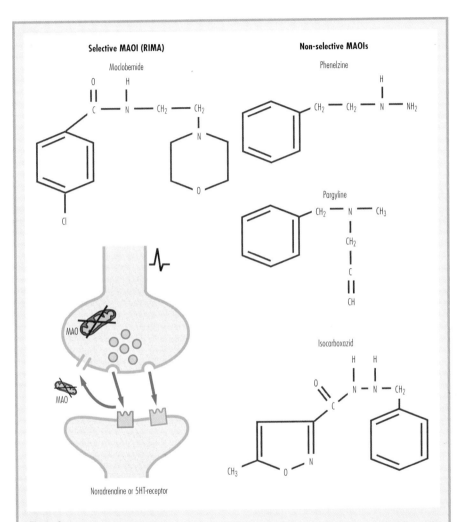

Figure 8
Action of MAOIs on monoamine function. Non-selective MAOIs are irreversible inhibitors of MAO. Thus any dietary amines, as well as endogenous amines, will not be metabolized. If dietary amines are present in high concentration (for example, beer, red wines, ripe cheeses, fermented meats, etc) they will displace noradrenaline from nerve terminals and cause hypertension. Reversible MAOI inhibitors (RIMAs) can be displaced in the wall of the gastrointestinal tract by dietary amines which are then metabolized and thus less likely to enter the blood and cause hypertension.

Figure 9
Action of SNRIs on monoamine reuptake. These drugs selectively block the reuptake of noradrenaline and serotonin but do not block adrenoceptors, H₁-receptors or cholinergic-1 receptors. The mechanism of action is, therefore, similar to that of TCAs without the adrenergic, histaminergic and cholinergic side-effects. (See Figure 10 for diagram of action).

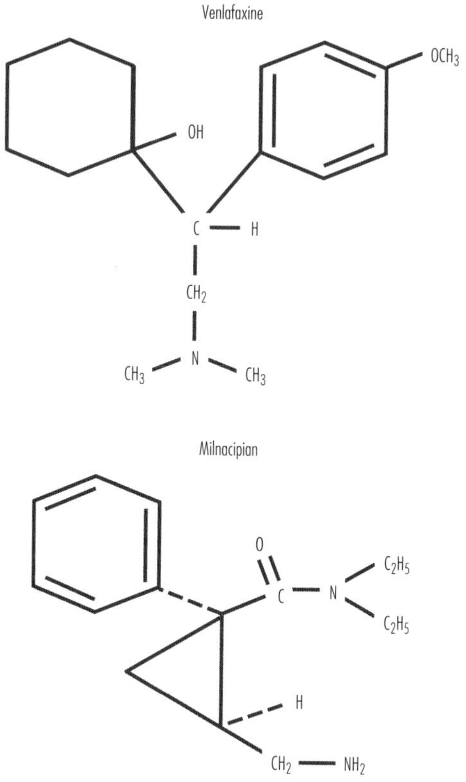

Venlafaxine

Milnacipian

The serotonin and noradrenaline uptake inhibitors (SNRIs)

These differ structurally from the TCAs and have no direct action on the muscarinic, histaminic or adrenergic receptors. Nevertheless, the side-effects listed in the next paragraph have been reported with venlafaxine. It seems probable that milnacipran will also cause some tachycardia and slight hypertension similar effects, although data are currently limited because the drug has only recently been launched in some European countries. With venlafaxine the side-effects appear to be dose dependent. Low therapeutic doses appear to affect the serotonergic system preferentially, whereas higher doses have an action on both the noradrenergic and the serotonergic systems.

The side-effects of low doses of venlafaxine are largely attributable to enhanced serotonergic function, and are similar to those seen after administration of the SSRIs, namely nausea, agitation, insomnia, sexual dysfunction. Higher therapeutic doses activate both the noradrenergic and the serotonergic systems and the side-effects include: hypertension, severe insomnia and agitation, nausea and headache. Hypercholesterolaemia has also been reported to occur in some patients receiving high doses of the drug.

Selective serotonin reuptake inhibitors (SSRIs)

The side-effects of the SSRIs are largely attributed to the enhanced serotonergic function, which results in the stimulation of the serotonin receptor in the spinal cord, gastrointestinal tract and brain. These side-effects are not related to the

antidepressant action of the drugs. As a consequence of the activation of serotonin receptors in the brain and the periphery, the following side-effects arise:

- *Neurological side-effects: agitation, akathisia, anxiety, insomnia, sexual dysfunction.*

- *Vascular side-effects: headache, migraine-like attacks.*

- *Gastrointestinal side-effects: nausea, vomiting, diarrhoea.*

Neurological side-effects

Many of the motor side-effects (for example, akathisia, agitation) appear to be initiated by excessive stimulation of the $5HT_2$-receptors in the serotonergic pathway which projects to the basal ganglia. It is postulated that the $5HT_2$-receptors inhibit the release of dopamine and thereby lead to a deficiency in the 'motor' neurotransmitter dopamine. This leads to akathisia (a form of motor restlessness) and agitation. The precipitation of extrapyramidal side-effects may also occur in some patients with Parkinson's disease who are being treated with L-dopa and concomitantly with an SSRI for depression. Caution should therefore always be exercised in treating the depressed state of such a patient with an SSRI or venlafaxine.

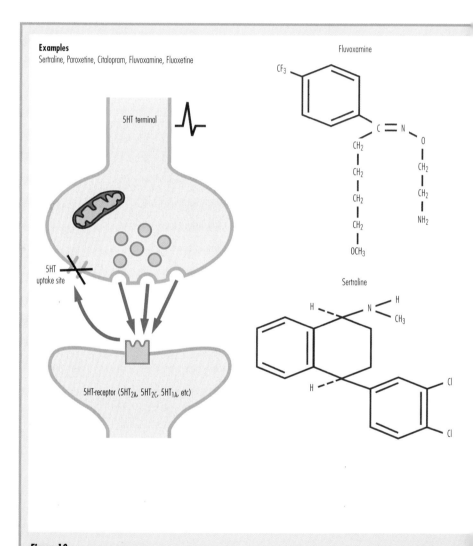

Figure 10
Action of SSRIs on serotonin reuptake. SSRIs have no direct action on 5HT-receptors or on other monoamine transmitters. Nefazodone also blocks 5HT reuptake but in addition blocks postsynaptic 5HT₂-receptors.

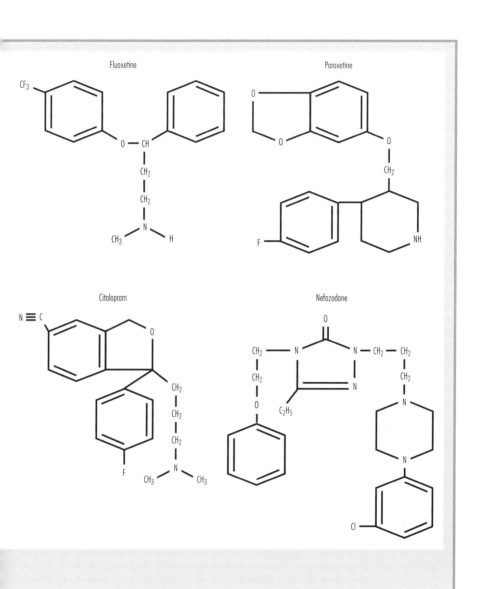

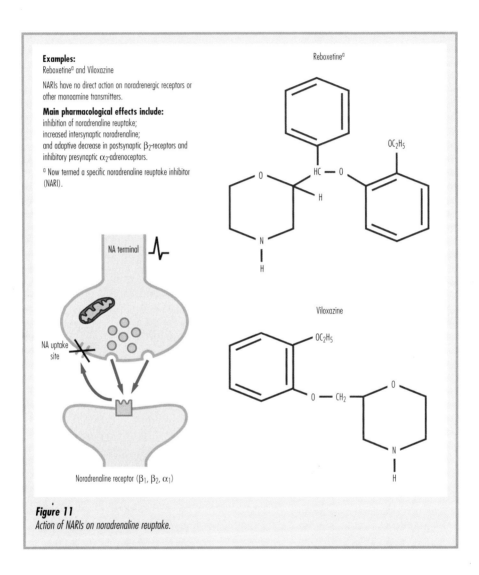

Examples:
Reboxetine[a] and Viloxazine

NARIs have no direct action on noradrenergic receptors or other monoamine transmitters.

Main pharmacological effects include:
inhibition of noradrenaline reuptake;
increased intersynaptic noradrenaline;
and adaptive decrease in postsynaptic β_2-receptors and inhibitory presynaptic α_2-adrenoceptors.

[a] Now termed a specific noradrenaline reuptake inhibitor (NARI).

Reboxetine[a]

Viloxazine

NA terminal

NA uptake site

Noradrenaline receptor (β_1, β_2, α_1)

Figure 11
Action of NARIs on noradrenaline reuptake.

Although the serotonin–dopamine inter-action is the most probable cause of the motor side-effects, recent research also indicates that some SSRIs (such as fluoxetine and fluvoxamine) sensitize the σ_2-receptors in the rubrocerebellar region

Figure 12
The tetracyclic antidepressants mianserin and mirtazapine on monoamine functions. Mianserin and mirtazapine are examples of dual action antidepressants. They enhance noradrenergic and serotonergic function by blocking the inhibitory α2-adrenoceptors on noradrenergic terminals and the α2-heteroceptors on serotonergic terminals. A diagram illustrating the proposed mechanism of action of mirtazapine is shown in **Figure 5**. Mirtazapine is more effective than mianserin in enhancing serotonergic function because it increases the firing rate of serotonergic neurons. Mianserin is less potent than mirtazapine in blocking postsynaptic serotonin receptors.

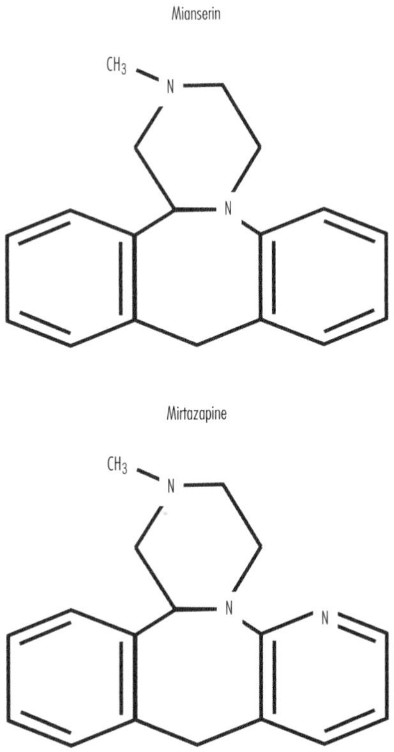

Mianserin

Mirtazapine

of the lower brain. The activation of these receptors has also been implicated in akathisia and agitation.

Anxiety frequently arises during the initial period of treatment with SSRIs, the frequency of this effect varying with the type of SSRI. Thus fluoxetine has been most frequently associated with anxiety, sertraline and paroxetine with a lower frequency, and citalopram and fluvoxamine are the least likely to be associated. These effects are usually of short duration (1–2 weeks) and largely remit after the onset of the antidepressant effect. It has been postulated that SSRI-induced anxiety, and occasionally panic attacks, arise as a consequence of excessive stimulation of the $5HT_2$ receptors which project from the raphe nucleus to the hippocampus and limbic cortex. After the desensitization of these receptors, following long-term administration of the SSRIs, these drugs exhibit an anxiolytic effect. Indeed, clinical trials show that the SSRIs (particularly the less alerting SSRIs such as fluvoxamine and citalopram) are equally effective to the anxiolytic benzodiazepines. In placebo-controlled studies, it is interesting that the SSRIs are more effective than the sedative TCAs (such as imipramine) in attenuating the anxiety symptoms, which are a common feature of depression.

Insomnia also frequently occurs in the initial stages of SSRI administration and is believed to occur as a result of the serotonergic-mediated activation of the cholinergic neurons in the lateral tegmental region of the brain-stem sleep centre. As a consequence, the slow wave sleep profile in particular is disrupted. It is postulated that nocturnal myoclonus, leading to an increased frequency of nocturnal awakenings, arises as a result of the disturbed sleep patterns. Bruxism (teeth grinding) during the night has also been reported to occur after chronic SSRI treatment, but the precise mechanism is currently uncertain.

Sexual dysfunction is a fairly common feature of the SSRIs and results in delayed ejaculation (or rarely impotence) in men and anorgasmia in women. The incidence is said to vary between 7 and 40% in male patients. The physiological basis of human sexual function is complex and poorly understood. Furthermore, it must be emphasized that, like anxiety, loss of libido is a core feature of depression. It is believed that loss of libido and poor sexual function are associated with a decreased activity of the mesolimbic dopamine pathways. The serotonergic system inhibits the dopaminergic system in this brain region, via the $5HT_2$ receptors, and thereby reduces the pleasure and arousal usually associated with sexual function. It is also interesting that the craving for drugs of abuse such as cocaine and amphetamine stimulants is rewarded by the release of dopamine from the mesolimbic system; those abusing such drugs often experience an orgasmic-like state. Thus, it has been postulated that the SSRIs, by inhibiting the doaminergic pathways, cause sexual dysfunction in both male and female patients. In addition, ejaculation and orgasm are associated with the descending serotonergic pathways from the brain stem to the spinal cord. Increased serotonin release, which occurs after the prolonged administration of an SSRI, thereby inhibits these components of sexual function.

Apart from changing to a non-serotonergic antidepressant, such as an NARI (for example, reboxetine), a TCA (for example, nortritpyline) or an MAOI (such as moclobemide), it is occasionally possible to reverse the sexual side-effects of an SSRI by administering a $5HT_1$-, $5HT_2$-receptor antagonist such as cyproheptadine or allowing 1 or 2 days of a drug holiday by stopping the SSRI. Drug holidays are of course limited to the shorter half-life SSRIs such as sertraline, fluvoxamine, citalopram or paroxetine. Alternatively, nefazodone, the SSRI with $5HT_2$-receptor antagonist action, may be used because the sexual side-effects of this drug are said to be much lower than those of the conventional SSRIs. It is theoretically possible that combining an SSRI with mianserin or mirtazapine may also reduce the incidence of sexual side-effects and even bring forward the onset of the antidepressant effect.

Not all the effects of the SSRIs on sexual function are negative, however. There is anecdotal evidence in the literature that low acute doses of the shorter-acting SSRIs can be used to treat premature ejaculation, which is accepted as a very common problem, not only in those patients with depression or anxiety.

Vascular side-effects

Headache, and migraine, probably arise as a consequence of the excessive stimulation by serotonin of the $5HT_{1D}$-receptors located on the walls of the cerebral vessels. After prolonged administration of the SSRIs, however, the sensitivity of these receptors decreases and such side-effects are therefore largely related to the initial period of treatment.

Gastrointestinal side-effects

Nausea, and occasionally vomiting, are common side-effects of all the SSRIs, and to a lesser extent of venlafaxine and nefazodone. These effects are the result of stimulation of the $5HT_3$-receptors located in the vomiting centre, but they also result from stimulation of the $5HT_3$-receptors located in the intestine. Increased activity of the $5HT_3$-receptors in the intestine also leads to activation of the intestinal smooth muscle, leading to diarrhoea and occasionally gastrointestinal cramps. It is not surprising to find that anorexia and loss of appetite occasionally occur in patients taking SSRIs. This is most probably associated with the nausea, but may also be attributed to the influence of the increase in the serotonergic input to the hypothalamus.

Monoamine oxidase inhibitors (MAOIs)

The major problems with the older irreversible inhibitors of monoamine oxidase (MAO), such as phenelzine, isocarboxazid and tranylcypromine, arises from their interaction with primary amines, such as tryptamine, contained in the diet. In brief, all primary amines found in the diet are usually metabolized by MAO contained in the wall of the gastrointestinal tract. Inhibition by MAOIs therefore allows the passage of these amines into the blood, from where they can be transported by the noradrenaline uptake sites into sympathetic nerve terminals. This can result in an abrupt displacement of noradrenaline from its storage vesicles and a non-neuronal release of the amine onto the α_1- and β_1-receptors on the blood vessel walls and the myocardium. The increased cardiac output, combined with the sudden hypertension resulting from the vasoconstriction of the small blood vessels, may therefore cause a cardiovascular crisis and even a stroke. The development of the reversible and selective MAOIs (reversible inhibitors of MAO (or RIMAs) such as moclobemide) largely overcame those problems because an excess of dietary amines in the gastrointestinal tract removes the MAOI from the MAO and allows the enzyme to catabolize the dietary amines. In the brain, and peripheral sympathetic nervous system, the MAOI is still inhibited by the reversible MAOI, allowing the RIMA to continue to function.

Providing the patient is compliant and carefully monitors the type of foods consumed, however, all the MAOIs have a valuable role to play as second-line antidepressants, particularly in those patients with atypical depression characterized by weight gain and hypersomnia, and those with panic attacks.

The main side-effects of the irreversible MAOIs are hypotension, insomnia and occasionally sexual dysfunction. Although the cause of insomnia and sexual dysfunction can be explained by the enhanced serotonergic function (see side-effects of the SSRIs), the hypotensive effect is postulated to occur as a consequence of the increase in the concentration of dopamine, which acts as an inhibitory transmitter in the sympathetic ganglia. By preventing the catabolism of dopamine in the ganglia, the dopamine concentration increases, thereby leading to a reduction in the functional activity of the main excitatory transmitter acetylcholine. Ganglionic transmission is reduced and the sympathetic tone likewise decreased, which can lead to a dramatic drop in blood pressure in some patients.

Atypical antidepressants and noradrenergic and specific serotonergic antidepressants (NASSAs)

The atypical antidepressants are exemplified by mianserin, mirtazapine and trazodone. The main side-effect of these three antidepressants is sedation as a result of their potent antihistaminic actions. Weight gain is also a problem and may be attributed partly to the antihistaminic action of these drugs.

Mianserin was the first novel antidepressant to be developed after the introduction of the TCAs and non-selective MAOIs. Its main clinical advantage lay in its lack of anticholinergic side-effects, but the hypotensive action (caused by blockade of α_1-adrenoceptors) and potent antihistaminic effects (resulting in drowsiness and sedation) limited its widespread application. Rare cases of agranulocytosis (and blood dyscrasias) also caused concern. Mirtazapine, a structural analogue of mianserin, lacks the α_1-receptor antagonist effect but is still likely to cause sedation and drowsiness. Reversible white blood cell disorders have been reported to occur after the administration of mirtazapine according to the product information presented by the manufacturer but the frequency of such effects would appear to be low according to the published literature.

Trazodone has many of the side-effects associated with mianserin. In addition, it has been found to cause priapism in elderly male patients which has restricted its use in elderly male depressives.

Summary

Many of the side-effects of antidepressants are attributable to the actions of the drugs on receptors that are not associated with their antidepressant actions (such as the adrenoceptors, muscarinic receptors and histamine receptors). However, some side-effects are an inevitable consequence of activation of the serotonergic system and include the neurological, sexual and gastrointestinal side-effects. Such effects occur with the SSRIs, SNRIs and MAOIs. Dietary interactions are largely confined to the non-selective MAOIs.

Withdrawal problems with antidepressants

Although there is no evidence to imply that any currently available antidepressants are drugs of abuse, there is evidence to show that the abrupt withdrawal of most classes of antidepressants is associated with untoward effects. For example, it is well known that the abrupt withdrawal of a TCA results in the following syndromes: gastrointestinal and general somatic distress, anxiety and agitation, sleep disturbance, tremor, movement disorders and, occasionally, paradoxical activation of mania. Many of these symptoms could be attributed to the re-emergence of the underlying symptoms of anxiety–depression, although the fact that they may emerge a few days after discontinuation of the medication also suggests that they are a consequence of drug withdrawal. This has led to the British National Formulary issuing the following warning.

> *Gastrointestinal symptoms of nausea, vomiting and anorexia, accompanied by headache, giddiness, 'chills', insomnia and sometimes hypomania, panic anxiety and extreme motor restlessness, may occur if an antidepressant, particularly an MAOI, is stopped suddenly after regular administration for 8 weeks or more. Reduction in dosage should preferably be carried out over a period of about 4 weeks.*

Although the frequency of spontaneous reporting of the withdrawal effects of the TCAs and MAOIs is very low, a proportionally larger number of cases of problems with withdrawal from the SSRIs have been reported in recent years. This may be the result of an improvement in the frequency of reporting the adverse effects of all drugs or of the higher incidence of withdrawal effects after the abrupt cessation of treatment with some SSRIs. Of the five SSRIs marketed in Europe, the percentage of withdrawal problems reported to the Committee on Safety of Medicines by 1997 was 6% for fluoxetine and sertraline, and about 1% for fluvox-

amine, citalopram and nefazodone. The SSRI that caused the most frequent withdrawal effects (84% of the total) was paroxetine. By comparison, the SNRI antidepressant venlafaxine only caused 2% of the withdrawal effects of antidepressants reported. The main withdrawal effects reported for venlafaxine were dizziness, sweating, nausea, insomnia, tremor and confusion. These adverse effects usually start within a few days of abrupt withdrawal and largely resolve on reinstating the drug. Thus, to avoid such unpleasant effects, it is generally recommended that no SSRI should be withdrawn abruptly.

Summary

*All antidepressants produce withdrawal symptoms of a varying severity after their prolonged administration. These symptoms frequently include insomnia, gastric disturbances, anxiety and dizziness. Although some of these symptoms may be associated with a re-emergence of the underlying depression, the fact that they often occur shortly after drug withdrawal and remit on readministering the antidepressant suggest that they result from antidepressant withdrawal. For this reason, it is always advisable to withdraw a antidepressant slowly or over a period of several weeks by tapering down the dose (**Table 10**).*

Table 10
Relationship between changes in neurotransmitter receptor function, antidepressant action and predictable side-effects.

TCAs

Inhibition of noradrenaline and serotonin reuptake leads to antidepressant effect

Inhibition of muscarinic (M_1) receptors leads to blurred vision, dry mouth, tachycardia, delayed micturition, precipitation of glaucoma

Inhibition of histamine (H_1) receptors leads to sedation, drowsiness and (possibly) weight gain

Inhibition of α_1-adrenoceptors leads to orthostatic hypertension

All these side-effects are particularly pronounced in the elderly patient

MAOIs

Reduction in monoamine metabolism leads to antidepressant effect

Inhibition of cholinergic transmission in sympathetic ganglia (caused by enhanced dopaminergic function) leads to orthostatic hypotension

Increased serotonergic transmission in brain stem leads to insomnia

Increased serotonergic transmission in mesolimbic dopaminergic system and in spinal neurons leads to sexual dysfunction

SSRIs

Inhibition of serotonin reuptake leads to antidepressant effect

Inhibition of dopaminergic transmission by increased serotonergic function in basal ganglia leads to movement disorders

Increased serotonergic activity in hippocampus and hippocampus and limbic cortex leads to anxiety

Increased serotonergic transmission in brain stem leads to insomnia

Increased serotonergic transmission in the mesolimbic doipaminergic system and in spinal neurons leads to sexual dysfunction

Stimulation of $5HT_3$-receptors in vomiting centre and gastrointestinal tract leads to nausea, vomiting, diarrhoea

Trazodone

Inhibition of serotonin reuptake and block of postsynaptic $5HT_2$-receptors leads to antidepressant effect

Inhibition of histamine (H_1) receptors leads to sedation, drowsiness orthostatic hypotension

Inhibition of α_1-adrenoceptors leads to orthostatic hypotension

M-chlorophenyl piperazine (MCPP) metabolite leads to anxiety in high doses

Cont'd.

Mianserin

Inhibition of presynaptic α_2-adrenoceptors and postsynaptic $5HT_2$-receptors leads to antidepressant effect

Inhibition of histamine (H_1) receptors leads to drowsiness, sedation and (possibly) weight gain

Inhibition of α_1-adrenoceptors leads to orthostatic hypotension

Mirtazapine

Inhibition of presynaptic α_2-adrenoceptors and postsynaptic $5HT_2$-receptors, indirect stimulation of $5HT_{1A}$-receptors leads to antidepressant and anxiolytic effects

Inhibition of histamine (H_1) receptors leads to drowsiness, sedation and (possibly) weight gain

Inhibition of $5HT_3$-receptors leads to lack of gastrointestinal tract effects (nausea, diarrhoea, etc)

NARIs, for example, reboxetine

Inhibition of noradrenaline reuptake leads to antidepressant effect

Enhanced peripheral sympathetic function may occasionally lead to tachycardia

Enhanced central sympathetic function leads to insomnia

SNRIs, for example, venlafaxine

Inhibition of noradrenaline and serotonin reuptake (compare TCAs) leads to antidepressant effect

Low therapeutic doses primarily increase serotonergic function leading to nausea, agitation, sexual dysfunction and insomnia (compare side-effects of SSRIs)

Intermediate to high doses leads to hypertension, resulting from increased sympathetic activity severe insomnia, agitation, nausea and headache caused by SSRI-related side-effects. An enhanced dopaminergic effect may contribute to the severe nausea

Nefazodone

Inhibition of serotonin reuptake and block of postsynaptic $5HT_2$-receptor leads to antidepressant effect

Weak inhibitor of noradrenaline reuptake and α_1-adrenoceptors leads to negligible effect on blood pressure

Increased serotonergic transmission in brain stem leads to insomnia

M-Chlorophenyl piperazine metabolite (MCPP) leads to anxiety in high doses

Drug interactions of potential clinical importance

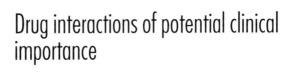

More than 90% of the drugs administered to a patient are metabolized in the liver. Interactions between drugs can then arise either if two or more drugs compete for the same enzyme system, which could become saturated with the drug substrate, or if one of the drugs inhibits the liver enzyme and therefore prevents metabolism of the second drug.

Although many drug interactions have remained largely of theoretical interest because significant problems do not arise in clinical practice, there are occasions when drugs with a low therapeutic index are given in combination with drugs that inhibit their metabolism. For example, some of the SSRIs such as fluoxetine are potent inhibitors of some of the cytochrome P450 (Cyt P450) isozymes that metabolize the TCAs. Concurrent administration of a TCA with fluoxetine causes a three- to fourfold increase in the plasma concentration of the TCA which could lead to severe cardiotoxic effects. Thus knowledge of potential drug interactions is essential for good clinical practice.

Genetic and environmental factors that influence drug metabolism

The activities of many of the main groups of enzymes that metabolize drugs, the Cyt P450 isozymes, which can be inhibited, include such commonly used drugs as cimetidine and carbamazepine, as well as herbal medicines, environmental toxins (such as polycyclic hydrocarbons, insecticides and herbicides), steroid and sex hormones, alcohol, caffeine, tobacco smoke, vegetables such as members of the cabbage family, and even diets that are high or low in protein. Those substances that can inhibit the Cyt P450 isozymes can act as reversible or irreversible inhibitors. If they irreversibly inhibit the Cyt P450 system, their effect on drug metabolism will be prolonged because new enzymes must be synthesized before metabolism can return to normal. Drugs such as the barbiturates can have the opposite effect on the Cyt P450 system and actually enhance the activity of the enzymes by causing an increased

synthesis of enzyme protein. This occurs as a result of increased gene transcription.

In the case of enzyme induction, any drug that is metabolized by the Cyt P450 enzyme system is likely to be metabolized more rapidly and therefore have a shorter duration of action than normal.

Genetic polymorphism refers to the differences between individuals in their ability to metabolize drugs. Over 25 years ago, it was reported that the steady-state plasma concentration of nortriptyline was related to the genetic composition of the patient. Thus homozygous twins had similar blood nortriptyline concentrations after receiving the same dose of the drug, whereas heterozygous twins showed considerable variations in the blood concentration of the drug. It is now evident that many of the liver enzymes involved with drug metabolism exhibit genetic polymorphism, and this gives rise to subgroups in the population that differ in their ability to metabolize drugs. For example, individuals with deficient metabolism are known as poor metabolizers and are therefore more likely to accumulate an antidepressant than those with normal metabolism. Conversely, others may be fast metabolizers of an antidepressant and will therefore have a poorer clinical response to the standard dose of an antidepressant that is metabolized by the Cyt P450 system. Major problems are only likely to arise, however, if the drug administered concurrently with an inhibitor of one of the Cyt P450 isozymes has a low therapeutic index (for example, a TCA, a phenothiazine neuroleptic or an antiarrhythmic drug.).

Of the 30 or so isozymes that make up the Cyt P450 system in the liver and that bring about the oxidative metabolism of drugs, four are particularly important for

the metabolism of psychoactive drugs; these are known as 1A2, 2C, 2D6 and 3A4. The isozymes that metabolize different classes of antidepressants, are summarized in *Table 11*.

There is a probability of significant drug interactions when an inhibitor of one of the Cyt P450 isozymes is given together with a drug that is metabolized by that isozyme. Some of the most important drug interactions that might arise in such circumstances are given in *Table 12*.

In addition to the possible metabolic interactions outlined above, consideration should always be given to drug–protein

Table 11
Metabolism of antidepressants by liver enzymes.

Cyt P450 isozyme	Antidepressant metabolized
IA2	TCAs: amitriptyline, imipramine, clomipramine – demethylated
2D6	TCAs: imipramine, amitriptyline, nortriptyline – hydroxylated paroxetine, venlafaxine

Specific isozymes responsible for the metabolism of fluoxetine, sertraline, fluvoxamine, nefazodone, trazodone are unknown. These drugs have high affinities for the Cyt P450 isozymes and inhibit them.

Table 12
Drug interactions that could occur as a result of the inhibition of some Cyt P450 isozymes.

Cyt P450 isozyme	Substrates	Inhibitors
IA2	Phenacetin Caffeine[a] Theophylline[a] Haloperidol[a] TCAs	Fluvoxamine (Venlafaxine, nefazodone, mirtazapine)
2C9	Diazepam[a] TCAs Warfarin Phenytoin Tolbutamide[a]	Fluoxetine Fluvoxamine Sertraline (Venlafaxine, mirtazapine)
2D6	Haloperidol Thioridazine Perphenazine[a] Clozapine Risperidone TCAs[a] Paroxetine Venlafaxine Codeine β Blockers Type 1C antiarrhythmics[a] Verapamil	Fluoxetine Norfluoxetine Paroxetine Sertraline (Venlafaxine, fluvoxamine, mirtazapine)

3A4	TCAs	Sertraline
	Triazolam[a]	Fluoxetine
	Alprazolam[a]	Fluvoxamine
	Midazolam	Nefazodone
	Carbamazepine[a]	(Venlafaxine, paroxetine, mirtazapine)
	Terfenadine	
	Quinidine	
	Lignocaine	

[a] *Possible interactions of clinical significance. Antidepressants shown in brackets inhibit these enzymes only in high concentrations and are therefore unlikely to present major problems.*

binding interactions. Clearly, two highly protein-bound (>95%) drugs that are attached to the same binding site on the same plasma protein might interact if given together. However, so far this possi- bility does not appear to have any clinical significance with regard to second-genera- tion antidepressants, many of which are highly protein bound (80–90%).

Summary

The occurrence of serious drug interactions involving antidepressants can be reduced by knowing which drugs are likely to be inhibited by an anti- depressant and reducing the dose of the inhibited drug and/or the initial dose of the antidepressant. Good therapeutic practice demands the moni- toring of pharmacodynamic effects at all times, particularly in those subpopulations of depressed patients such as elderly people or those with hepatic dysfunction or a history of alcoholism which could be associated with liver damage. It is not recommended to combine an SSRI with a TCA because of the potential for a marked increase in the plasma concentrations, resulting in possible cardiotoxicity.

Role of serotonin in depression

7

Serotonin and noradrenaline have both been implicated
in the aetiology of depression. Recently the development
of novel non-benzodiazepine anxiolytic drugs, such as
buspirone has shown that a subpopulation of serotonin
receptors, in particular the $5HT_{1A}$-receptors, is implicated
in anxiety disorders. To add to the complexity of the role
of serotonin in the pathology of anxiety disorders, there
is clinical evidence that impulsive behaviour as exhibited
by patients with obsessive–compulsive disorder, alcoholism, compulsive gambling and bulimia, probably involves
a defect in central serotoninergic transmission. Whether
serotonin is the primary cause of impulsive behaviour
and depression, or whether it acts indirectly to modulate
the activity of other neurotransmitters, is currently
unclear.

Biochemical aspects

Serotonin is an indoleamine that is synthesized in the
brain and periphery from L-tryptophan. The main
pathway leading to the synthesis and catabolism of
serotonin is illustrated in *Figure 13*.

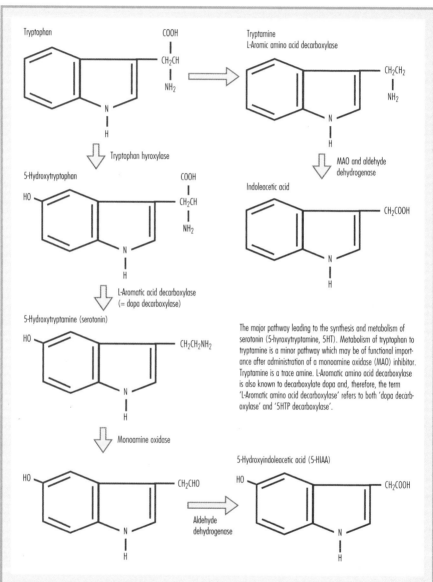

Figure 13
Main pathway leading to the synthesis of serotonin.

L-tryptophan is the dietary precursor of the endogenous indoleamine serotonin and tryptamine. About 85% of tryptophan is bound to the serum proteins. This implies that only about 15% of the tryptophan is available for transport across the blood–brain barrier where it enters the amino acid pool for protein, peptide and indoleamine synthesis. In the periphery, the free form of tryptophan also acts as the precursor of serotonin in the platelets and enterochromaffin cells. It can be metabolized in the liver by the kynurenine pathway. The activity of this pathway may be induced by steroidal hormones, including oestrogens. By enhancing the liver catabolism of tryptophan, it has been suggested that the depressive episodes, which sometimes occur in those taking the high-oestrogen contraceptive pill, may be attributed to a decreased synthesis of serotonin in the brain as a result of a decrease in the availability of free tryptophan. The liver kynurenine pathway can also be altered by endogenous glucocorticoids, some components of the diet and by changes in the circadian rhythm, all of which may play a role in modulating serotonin synthesis in the brain.

The importance of tryptophan as a precursor of serotonin may be illustrated by the changes in mood of the depressed patient who is in remission but maintained on an SSRI and who has been temporarily deprived of L-tryptophan by the administration of a tryptophan-free drink containing an excess of other essential amino acids. It has been found that a depressive episode is rapidly precipitated; experimental studies demonstrate that the release of serotonin in the cortex is dramatically reduced under these conditions. The rapid onset of the depressive episode does not occur in all patients, however, but appears to be particularly prevalent in those patients who are in remission but maintained on SSRI antidepressants. It is currently difficult to understand how the symptoms of depression in these patients can be precipitated so rapidly after the administration of a tryptophan-deficient diet and yet the SSRI antidepressants take several weeks to ameliorate the symptoms. Could it be possible that the rapid onset of depression occurs by the same underlying mechanism, which is the basis for the rapid onset of the antidepressant effect after sleep deprivation therapy? There are several reports showing that sleep deprivation therapy results in an alleviation in the mood of the depressed patient within a few days. However, this beneficial effect is not sustained. Perhaps this could be associated with temporary changes in amine neurotransmitter receptor function, whereas a sustained antidepressant response only occurs when there are changes in the gene expression of the processes that underlie the abnormal neurotransmitter synthesis, release and metabolism.

Mechanism of action of SSRIs

Evidence has already been summarized *(see Chapter 4)* to indicate that the serotonergic system is malfunctional in depression. In summary, it has been postulated that the SSRIs ultimately normalize central serotonergic neurotransmission by bringing about adaptive changes in the somatodendritic $5HT_{1A}$-(inhibitory) receptors and the postsynaptic $5HT_{2A}$-receptors. Serotonin release may also be facilitated by the desensitization of the $5HT_{1D}$-autoreceptors which normally reduce the release of the transmitter after their stimulation. Thus, it may be postulated that initially the SSRIs block the reuptake of serotonin in the raphe region where the serotonin transport sites are particularly dense. This increases the concentration of the transmitter in the vicinity of the somatodendritic $5HT_{1A}$-receptors. On stimulation, these inhibitory receptors reduce the release of serotonin from the terminal regions. Prolonged stimulation of the somatodendritic receptors leads to their desensitization and there is a consequent reduction in their inhibitory action on serotonin release from the nerve terminals.

This action, combined with the desensitization of the inhibitory $5HT_{1D}$-autoreceptors, thereby leads to an enhanced release of serotonin and a decrease in the density of the postsynaptic $5HT_{2A}$. Thus the mechanism of action of the SSRIs may be visualized as an adaptational balance between the inhibitory $5HT_{1A}/5HT_{1D}$-receptors and the postsynaptic $5HT_{2A}$-receptors. This process takes several weeks to become fully effective.

The possible mechanism of action of the SSRIs is summarized in *Figure 14*.

In addition to their well-established antidepressant action, the SSRIs are also of therapeutic value in the treatment of anxiety disorders. Whereas the antidepressant action of the SSRIs is postulated to result from the enhanced activity of the midbrain (raphe) to prefrontal cortex projection, it is hypothesized that the antiobsessive–compulsive disorder action

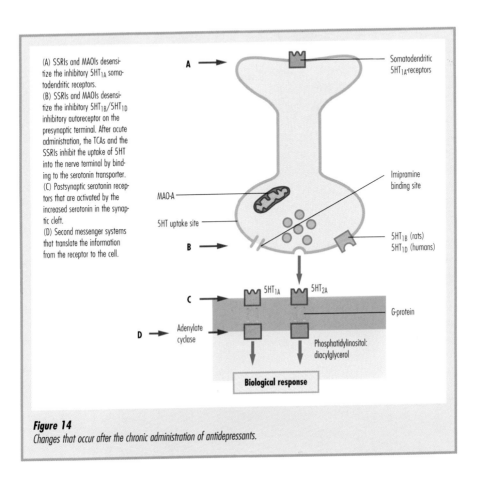

(A) SSRIs and MAOIs desensitize the inhibitory 5HT₁ₐ somatodendritic receptors.
(B) SSRIs and MAOIs desensitize the inhibitory 5HT₁ᵦ/5HT₁ᴅ inhibitory autoreceptor on the presynaptic terminal. After acute administration, the TCAs and the SSRIs inhibit the uptake of 5HT into the nerve terminal by binding to the serotonin transporter.
(C) Postsynaptic serotonin receptors that are activated by the increased serotonin in the synaptic cleft.
(D) Second messenger systems that translate the information from the receptor to the cell.

Figure 14
Changes that occur after the chronic administration of antidepressants.

of the SSRIs results from their disinhibitory effect of the serotonergic pathway from the midbrain (raphe) to the basal ganglia.

The well-established antipanic actions of the SSRIs appear to be the result of a disinhibition of the serotonergic pathway which extends from the midbrain raphe to the hippocampus and limbic cortex. Initially, the degree of anxiety in the patient may slightly increase but then, as a result of desensitization of the $5HT_{1A}/5HT_{1D}$ and $5HT_{2A}$-receptors, the antipanic effect becomes established after several weeks of treatment.

The antibulimic actions of the SSRIs are postulated to result from a disinhibition of the serotonergic pathway which projects from the midbrain raphe to the hypothalamus. This leads to the activation of the serotonin receptor which normalizes feeding behaviour in the bulimic patient.

The main serotonergic pathways, which are postulated to be involved in these actions (antidepressant, antiobsessive–compulsive disorder, antipanic and anti-bulimic) of the SSRIs, are summarized in *Figure 15*.

Neurological side-effects of SSRIs

Akathisia and agitation occasionally occur as side-effects of the SSRIs, and may arise as a consequence of the overstimulation of $5HT_{2A}$-receptors in the basal ganglia. However, experimental evidence suggests

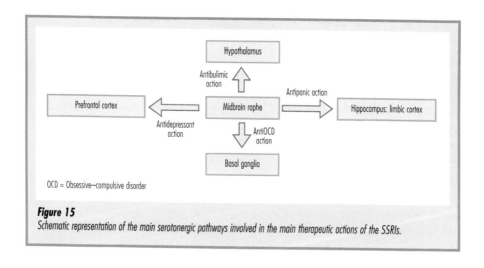

OCD = Obsessive–compulsive disorder

Figure 15
Schematic representation of the main serotonergic pathways involved in the main therapeutic actions of the SSRIs.

that the effects of the SSRIs on the $5HT_{2A}$-receptors are an indirect cause of akathisia and they are more likely to result from a reduction in the release of dopamine in the basal ganglia, in turn caused by the inhibitory effect of $5HT_{2A}$-heteroceptors. There is also experimental evidence to show that some SSRIs (such as fluoxetine and fluvoxamine) stimulate σ_2-receptors in the red nucleus which projects to the cerebellum. Stimulation of the σ-receptors may contribute to the akathisia. Whatever the mechanism for the movement disorders caused by the SSRIs, there is sufficient clinical evidence to suggest that care should be taken in administering this group of antidepressants to depressed patients with either Parkinson's disease or related movement disorders.

Other neurological side-effects of SSRIs which can result from the stimulation of serotonergic pathways in the brain, include anxiety and panic attacks; these are largely confined to the initial period of treatment with an SSRI and are assumed to result from the reduced release of serotonin from the hippocampal–limbic cortex region. Another side-effect is insomnia, which may arise in the initial few days of the SSRI treatment and is believed to be caused by the stimulation of $5HT_{2A}$-recep-

tors situated in the brain stem; this region projects to the cholinergic neurons in the lateral tegmental area, which probably regulate slow wave sleep. Disruption of the serotonergic–cholinergic balance may also be responsible for the occasional occurrence of nocturnal myoclonus.

Two other adverse effects of the SSRIs which appear to result from an enhanced serotonergic function, include sexual dysfunction and vomiting. Erectile dysfunction and delayed ejaculation frequently occur in the male patient after administration of an SSRI; the occurrence varies from less than 10% to over 40% according to the results of clinical trials. However, the incidence may be as high as 50%. In the female patient, anorgasmia has been reported but the incidence of this dysfunctional state is uncertain. One of the main problems in determining the relationship between the antidepressant treatment and the cause of the sexual dysfunction lies in the high incidence of sexual dysfunctional that occurs in depression, loss of libido being one of the common features of the condition.

It is hypothesized that SSRIs cause sexual dysfunction by reducing dopamine release from the mesocortical dopaminergic pathway. In this region of the brain, dopamine appears to act as a hedonic transmitter: its release causes a pleasurable effect. This, incidentally, is one of the main reasons why drugs of dependence are abused (because they release dopamine in the mesocortical region) and why the monoamine oxidise inhibitors (MAOIs) and dopaminergic activities of drugs such as buproprion do not cause sexual dysfunction.

Besides reducing libido in both male and female patients, the SSRIs can also enhance the brain stem–dorsal horn spinal pathway which inhibits ejaculation. Clearly the action of the SSRIs on sexual activity is complex, but the primary role played by the serotonergic system is the result of the beneficial action of non-specific serotonin receptor antagonists such as cyproheptadine which can reverse the SSRI-induced sexual dysfunction. However, the sedative effect of cyproheptadine (resulting from its antihistaminic action) precludes its routine use in this condition.

The brain-stem vomiting centre can be triggered by drugs that stimulate the $5HT_3$-receptors, which are situated on the chemoreceptor trigger zone. The slight nausea experienced by many patients early in treatment with an SSRI is attributed to stimulation of central and gastrointestinal $5HT_3$-receptors. Drugs that block the $5HT_3$-receptors, such as ondansetron and granisetron, antagonize the nauseant effects of the byproducts of cancer chemotherapy.

In addition to the direct effect of the SSRIs on the vomiting centre, there is also evidence that there is enhanced activity of the brain stem–hypothalamic pathway which mediates appetite and feeding behaviour. This could play a role in the anorexia and weight loss that occurs in some patients receiving an SSRI.

The main serotonergic pathways which appear to be used in the aetiology of the neurological side-effects of the SSRIs are summarized in *Figure 16*.

Extending the scope of therapeutic action of the SSRIs

There is preliminary evidence that the SSRIs are useful in the treatment of the following conditions:

- Pre-menstrual syndrome.
- Premature ejaculation.
- Fibromyalgia.
- Chronic pain syndromes.
- Negative symptoms of schizophrenia.

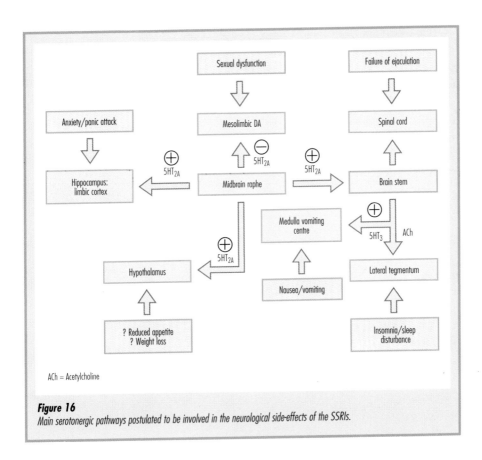

ACh = Acetylcholine

Figure 16
Main serotonergic pathways postulated to be involved in the neurological side-effects of the SSRIs.

However, none of these studies has been subject to double-blind placebo-controlled trials, and so the use of the SSRIs in these conditions rests largely on anecdotal reports.

With regard to the use of antidepressants in chronic pain, the only extensive placebo-controlled studies have involved the TCAs. The results of these studies suggest that antidepressants that inhibit the reuptake of both noradrenaline and serotonin are more effective than second-generation antidepressants such as mianserin, maprotiline, trazodone or zimelidine.

Although the precise mechanism by which the antidressants bring about their analgesic effects is unknown, it would appear that they exert them independently of their antidepressant effects. One possibility is that antidepressants that bring about chronic pain relief do so by activating opioid receptors directly or indirectly.

Summary

It would appear that the SSRIs are of little benefit in the treatment of pain associated with fibromyalgia or diabetic neuropathy, low back pain or rheumatic pain. There is no evidence that the SSRIs have any beneficial effects in treating either the positive or the negative systems of schizophrenia.

Role of noradrenaline in depression

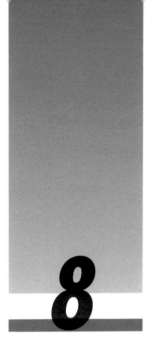

The monoamine hypothesis postulates that the primary cause of depression results from a malfunction of the noradrenergic and serotonergic systems in the brain. Despite the extensive studies of postmortem brains and body fluids from depressed patients and suicide victims, such studies have yielded mixed and sometimes confusing results. Nevertheless, there is evidence for a dysregulation of noradrenergic neurons in the cortical and hypothalamic areas of the depressed patient. For example, after the acute infusion of the α_2-adrenoceptor agonist clonidine into a depressed patient, the release of growth hormone from the pituitary gland is reduced. This response remains blunted even after recovery of the patient, which suggests that it could be a trait marker of the condition. Further evidence implicating an abnormality in noradrenergic function in depression arises from studies of the peripheral noradrenergic system. It has been shown that there is an increased release of noradrenaline in patients with major depression, which results in a decreased β-adrenoceptor responsiveness (as shown, for example, by a decreased responsiveness of the β-receptors on lymphocyte membranes to an isoprenaline challenge) and an increased activity of the α$_2$-adrenoceptors on the platelet membrane. This could be used as a model for the inhibitory presynaptic α$_2$-receptors which reduce noradrenaline release from the neurons.

There is accumulating evidence that the noradrenergic system modulates drive and motivation, whereas the serotonergic system modulates impulsiveness and mood. However, some of these functions, such as sleep disturbance and anxiety, overlap which is understandable in view of the close interrelationship of these two neuro-transmitter systems within the brain. Nevertheless, the noradrenergic system plays a key role in learning, memory, sleep, arousal and adaptation. It has been shown that, although the locus coeruleus, the main nucleus that controls noradren-ergic activity in the brain, is relatively quiescent during eating, sleeping and other behaviours, its activity increases whenever novel external stimuli are presented. Thus it would appear that noradrenaline plays an important role in the disturbance of vegetative function associated with affective and cognitive disorders, and anxiety. In addition, the locus coeruleus plays an essential role in adaptive and arousal responses. From experimental studies, it has been shown

that it fires in a phasic manner when the animal is subjected to a threatening stim-ulus. It would appear that this system becomes desynchronized in depression or when there is chronic exposure to stress, leading to malfunctioning of the central and peripheral sympathetic nervous systems.

Summary

There is evidence of altered central and sympathetic activity in the depressed patient, which may result from a primary malfunction of the main noradrenergic cell body area, the locus coeruleus. Effective antidepressant treatment may compensate for this.

Pharmacological properties of drugs that act on the brain's noradrenergic system

There was major advance in the treatment of depression with the development of the second generation of antidepressants; these combined the efficacy of the con-ventional TCAs with improved compliance as a result of the reduction in the adverse side-effects. Of the different classes of second-generation antidepressants that have been developed in the last 20 years, the SSRIs have achieved particular prominence. However, now they have been used extensively, it is becoming apparent that the SSRIs have adverse effects, particularly on the gastrointestinal tract and on sexual function, and many patients find this intolerable. Furthermore, there is growing evidence that the SSRIs are not as effective as the TCAs in the treatment of severe depression. This has led to the development of antidepressants such as venlafaxine and milnacipran which selectively inhibit the reuptake of noradrenaline and serotonin (but which lack the cardiotoxic effects of the TACs), and, more recently, a new generation of selective NARIs. As shown in *Table 13*, it is

Table 13
Effect of some antidepressants on neurotransmitter receptors in the brain tissue in vitro.

| | K_i (nmol/l) of adrenoceptors | | | | | |
	α_1	α_2	β	D_2	$5HT_1$	$5HT_2$
Representative SSRIs						
Fluoxetine	5990	>10 000	>5000	>10 000	>10 000	>1000
Sertraline	300	>5000	>5000	>5000	>10 000	>1000
SNRI						
Venlafaxine	>10 000	>10 000	>10 000	>10 000	>10 000	>7500
NARI						
Reboxetine	>10 000	>10 000	>10 000	>1000	>1000	>1000
Representative TCAs						
Amitriptyline	170	540	>5000	1200	1000	8
Clomipramine	38	3300	>5000	190	5200	63

K_i Values greater than 500 nmol/l imply that the drug would have no effect on the functional activitiy of the receptors in in vivo.
The inhibitory constant, K_i, is a measure of the potency of the drug in binding to the receptor. The lower the value, the higher the potency for the receptor.

apparent that none of the SNRIs, SSRIs or NARIs shows any affinity for the α- or β-adrenoceptors, the dopamine 2 (D_2-) receptor or the serotonin receptors, in contrast to the corresponding TCAs which have affinity for many of these receptor subtypes.

In contrast to the relative lack of effect of the second-generation antidepressants on the main neurotransmitter receptors implicated in depression, these drugs have a marked effect on the transporters for noradrenaline and serotonin in brain tissue. This is shown in *Table 14*.

Table 14
Inhibitory potency and relative selectivity of some antidepressants on monoamine uptake into brain tissue in vitro.

	Potency (nmol/l) of:		
	Inhibition of [^{3}H]5HT uptake	Inhibition of [^{3}H]noradrenaline uptake	Noradrenaline/5HT uptake inhibition ratio
SSRIs			
Fluoxetine	25	500	20
Sertraline	7.3	1400	190
SNRI			
Venlafaxine	39	213	5.4
NARI			
Reboxetine	1070	8.2	0.007
TCAs			
Amitriptyline	87	80	0.9
Clomipramine	7.4	100	13

Values greater than 500 nmol/l imply that the drug would have no effect on the functional activity of the transporter in vivo.

There are several classes of antidepressants that enhance noradrenergic function in the brain, but currently only the selective NARI, reboxetine, does so without affecting other uptake sites or neurotransmitter receptors. For example, the TCAs with a secondary amine side chain, such as desipramine, nortriptyline and protriptyline, and the modified TCA, maprotiline, show selectivity in inhibiting the noradrenaline transporter. However, their anticholinergic and cardiotoxic side-effects limit their use in many patients. Similarly the tetracyclic antidepressants, mianserin and mirtazapine, facilite noradrenaline release by blocking the inhibitory presynaptic α_2-adrenoceptors. However, these drugs also act on a number of serotonin receptors ($5HT_{1A}$, $5HT_2$, $5HT_3$). Of the cyclic antidepressants that are selective inhibitors of noradrenaline uptake, which include a number of drugs still in development (for example, tandamine, pirandamine, fluparoxan, talsupram and prindamine), only reboxetine has been marketed. In experimental studies, reboxetine has been shown to enhance noradrenaline release, presumably in blocking the inhibitory presynaptic α_2-receptors slightly, and to block noradrenaline reuptake selectively.

Reboxetine has been shown to be effective in several standard acute in vivo models used to detect antidepressant activity (such as the reversal of reserpine- and clonidine- induced hypothermia), and in the olfactory bulbectomized rat model of depression which is only sensitive to the antidepressant action of drugs after chronic administration. Reboxetine, like most effective antidepressants, was also shown to decrease the density of cortical β-adrenoceptors after chronic administration. A summary of the mechanism of action of reboxetine is shown in *Figure 11*.

In clinical studies, reboxetine has been shown to be an effective antidepressant in double-blind and placebo-controlled trials and to be equally effective with TCAs and some second-generation antidepressants. Any drug that selectively enhances noradrenergic function would be expected also to increase the peripheral sympathetic drive, which may cause an increase in blood pressure. Although acute healthy volunteer studies revealed slight increases in blood pressure, in short and long-term clinical studies changes in blood pressure were no more common on reboxetine than placebo The heart rate was slightly increased after reboxetine but desipramine had a more pronounced effect in increasing the heart rate when given to the volunteers in therapeutic doses (50–100 mg). In addition, reboxetine and desipramine shortened the recovery time of the light reflex response; these effects are consistent with the sympathomimetic effects of the drug, which are a consequence of the inhibition of noradrenaline reuptake inhibition. The slight reduction in the salivary volume found in these clinical studies probably reflects the enhancement of the noradrenaline-induced inhibition of central parasympathetic nuclei which follows the reduction in noradrenaline reuptake.

Summary

Reboxetine is the first of a series of NARI antidepressants which, in clinical trials, have been shown to be as effective as the TCAs and SSRIs, possibly with a reduced burden of side-effects and improved tolerability. Such drugs provide valuable tools for research into the role of noradrenaline in depression and help to extend the treatment of those depressed patients with low motivation and drive.

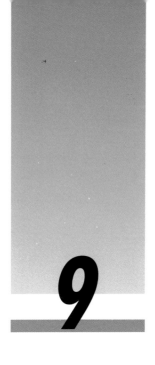

Strategies in treatment of resistant affective disorders

Individual antidepressants are conventionally said to work in two-thirds of the depressed patients who take them. It follows that there may be a significant proportion of non-responders to a first course of treatment. Subsequent interventions will depend on a strategic assessment of the probable risks and benefits. If treatment was initiated as a diagnostic exercise (does this individual have the kind of depression that is antidepressant responsive?), no further interventions may be called for. The more severe and classic the picture in terms of its 'biological' features, the greater the need to consider switching or combining pharmacological approaches. In either case a number of pharmacogenetic and pharmacokinetic factors should be considered. For the sake of simplicity, this chapter assumes that the unresponsive depressive state is not unresponsive primarily for reasons of personality or situation.

Pharmacogenetic considerations

Since the early 1960s it has been known that some people with mood disorders respond selectively to monoamine oxidase inhibitors (MAOIs), for instance, and others to TCAs. This seems to be genetically based. Where there is a history of exclusive response to MAOIs there is a likelihood that other family members will also be MAOI, rather than TCA, responders. The TCAs, which were used in these early studies by Rees and Pare, were drugs that also blocked reuptake of serotonin 5HT). The probability is therefore that, although most people with depressive disorders respond to any antidepressant, there is a proportion of people who respond selectively to either 5HT reuptake inhibition or to drugs that are active on the catecholaminergic system. A first step, therefore, in treatment-resistant mood disorders is to consider whether an individual who is currently taking an MAOI or a drug selective for noradrenergic systems, such as desipramine, lofepramine or reboxetine, should be switched to a drug active on the 5HT system or vice versa.

The rationale for such a switch is significantly increased if it appears that the individual has side-effects from the treatment. One good reason to suspect that an individual will be less likely to respond to an SSRI is if that individual has become more anxious on treatment. In this case, there is not so much a selective response to one group of agents as a failure to respond to another group; this failure results partly from the adverse effects caused by that group of agents in that particular individual.

Pharmacokinetic factors

Treatment may be complicated if it is being given together with an oral contraceptive, hormone replacement therapy, an analgesic or other agents, which may compete for plasma protein binding *(see Chapter 6)*. This can lead either to displacement of the antidepressant from its binding sites or to an increase in the amount of plasma protein available with the result that less antidepressant is available. In general any concomitant use of hormonal preparations requires an increased dose of antidepressant to maintain effective brain levels. When there is no response to the antidepressant, the co-administration of other compounds should be considered as a possible complicating factor either for these reasons or by virtue of interactions at target receptor sites. Indeed, any agents that are being co-administered should be considered as possible contributors to the depressive state, either as precipitants or as maintaining factors.

The role of the cytochrome P450 system and possible interactions at this locus have been considered in **Chapter 6**. In addition to interactions, there is also the possibility of up to 5–10% of individuals having significantly lower levels of one of the key cytochrome P450 enzymes. There are indications that up to 10% of non-responsiveness to neuroleptics may stem from factors such as this. Management approaches in the case of neuroleptics involves greatly reducing the dose to 10–20% of normal levels, for example, a dose of chlorpromazine may need to be reduced to 50 mg/day. There are no data linking non-response to antidepressants with these enzyme deficiencies, although there are large amounts of data that link non-response with enzyme deficiencies induced by the co-administration of other agents active on cytochrome enzyme systems. When it is possible to establish cytochrome genotypes at a biochemistry laboratory, this should be considered. By checking antidepressant blood levels there may be an indication of what is happening through revelation of high or low levels which are normally associated only with interference from competing agents.

Physical state

A wide range of physical states can trigger or maintain depressive disorders. Of these, the most notable are disturbances, of the thyroid and adrenal gland. Other states include a variety of occult carcinomas, in particular carcinoma of the pancreas. In elderly people, vascular lesions have a significant association with depressive states that are likely to be unresponsive to conventional approaches. Another trigger is those parkinsonian-like states that are currently subsumed under the heading Multiple System Atrophy *(Table 15)*. For these reasons, all treatment-resistant states will at some point require a thorough physical evaluation.

Treatment options

Option 1

Based on the above, and assuming that no physical diseases or pharmacokinetic

Table 15
Common physical disorders associated with depression.

1 Hypothyroidism
2 Cushing's disease and other disturbances of the hypothalamic–pituitary axis
3 Carcinoma, especially of the pancreas
4 Cardiac disorders – see ***Chapter 11***
5 Neurological disorders:
   (a) post stroke emotionalism
   (b) multi-infarct states
   (c) parkinsonian spectrum disorders

factors are contributing to non-response, the first option is to switch from an antidepressant of one class to one of another class.

Option 2

This strategy is to consider lithium augmentation, which was first introduced in Edinburgh and Norway in the early 1970s, but has since become known as the 'Newcastle cocktail'. The Newcastle version involves giving the combination of phenelzine, L-tryptophan and lithium; alternative versions involve the use of clomipramine, L-tryptophan and lithium. In the case of lithium augmentation, the early stories of 100% recovery rates occurring within hours of combining lithium with any other antidepressant appear to be unfounded. Less than 50% of the individuals who do not respond to treatment

can be expected to respond to these kinds of regimen and the response could take up to a month.

Option 3

A further strategy is to add mianserin or mirtazapine to either a TCA, MAOI or SSRI. This strategy, developed by Per Bech, appears to be particularly potent for severe depressive disorders. In many cases it brings about responses when the individual agents have not been effective. These combinations may also produce a reduction in the burden of side-effects rather than any increase predicted as a result of adding in a further psychotropic agent. Given similarities to mianserin in the receptor profiles, a comparable case can be made for adding trimipramine to an original front-line treatment.

Option 4

Another option is the addition of an anticonvulsant to the treatment regimen. The best known agents for this are carbamazepine and sodium valproate. Their primary use is in bipolar mood disorders, particularly atypical bipolar mood disorders that have proved difficult to stabilize, although there is considerable evidence that they also have a use in intractable recurrent unipolar disorders. More recently, the newly introduced anticonvulsants lamotrigine and gabapentin have been used in these areas, with early indications that the results could be promising.

Option 5

If the above regimens fail, it is worth considering the use of an antipsychotic. Most antipsychotics have at some point been subjected to placebo-controlled clinical trials in affective disorders, for example, haloperidol, thioridazine, sulpiride, flupenthixol. In general the reduction in tension provided by these agents could be useful in many mood disorders, and there is supportive evidence for this. As these agents retard psychomotor functions, they should be less useful in cases of melancholia which appears to be the case, although the addition of standard antipsychotics to antidepressant regimens is indicated in the treatment of depressive disorders that are overlaid with delusions.

There is also a good case for the addition of one of the newer atypical antipsychotics to otherwise refractory cases; this includes clozapine, quetiapine, sertindole, olanzapine, ziprasidone or amisulpiride. The stories of dramatic responses to clozapine achieved in extremely complex and severe clinical cases possibly owes something to its beneficial effects on intractable and complex mood disorders that are overlaid with a range of psychotic features, which often give rise to the diagnosis of a schizophrenic or schizoaffective disorder. In this group of patients there is at least anecdotal evidence of response to the other newer atypical antipsychotics.

Options 6

Electroconvulsive treatment (ECT) still remains the treatment that is considered to be most potent in refractory depressive disorders of biological origin. Rates of responsiveness of up to 90% can be expected in melancholic and delusional types of depression. There is therefore a temptation to resort to ECT in any nonresponsive condition. This temptation should be resisted unless there are clear indications of prior responses to ECT by the individual or other members of the family. There is a high risk of memory impairment in individuals with personality-based types of depression and accordingly, failure to respond to treatment increases the risk of injuring both the individual and the reputation of the treatment.

The treatment of recurrences

Primary care physicians are often bombarded with recommendations that treatment should continue for 6–12 months, or even longer, to reduce rates of relapse. These figures are taken in the main from hospitalized patients, and it is not clear how they should be translated into primary care. In general the briefer the depressive disorder, the less complicated is the response to treatment, the more clearly the individual returns to his norm, the less the need for a lengthy treatment.

The current conventional view, with regard to severe and recurrent types of depression, is that antidepressant therapy may induce a remission rather than a cure *(see Figure 17)*. In this case, treatment may need to be extended for months or even years until a proper cure supervenes. In these circumstances too early discontinuation of treatment will lead to a relapse – a re-emergence of the original disorder. In those cases where treatment does more

than induce a remission, future episodes are termed recurrences. For a cure to be achieved in a disorder that is liable to recur, prophylactic treatment with lithium, sodium valproate or carbamazepine may need to be considered. When remissions occur, adjunctive therapy may be indicated to bring about a more complete resolution of the disorder. In these cases adjunctive therapy may need to include psychotherapeutic or behavioural approaches or an appraisal of the patient's psychosocial situation.

In recent years recurrences have become more complex with recognition that, in a proportion of cases, antidepressants may be associated with discontinuation syndromes. If an apparently well patient appears to develop symptoms within hours or days of discontinuing treatment and, in particular, if this resolves within hours of reinstituting the original treatment, this is a discontinuation syndrome rather than a new illness episode. The management of such syndromes depends on the nature of the provoking agent. Combination treatments involving antidepressants and neuroleptics, such as tranylcypromine and trifluoperazine (parstelin), fluphenazine and nortriptyline (Motival) or amitriptyline (Triptafen) and fluphenazine, have been particularly likely to cause such problems.

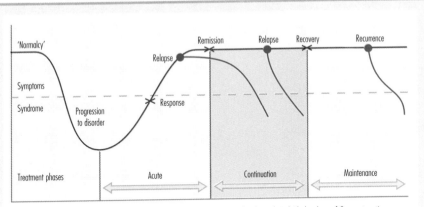

Response: the point at which an improvement of sufficient magnitude is observed rendering the individual no longer fully symptomatic.
Remission: a temporary cessation in the symptoms of depression.
Relapse: a return of the symptoms that satisfy the full syndromal criteria, occurring before the end of a 'natural' episode of depression.
Recovery: a return to a condition of normalcy.
Recurrence: the appearance of a new episode of a major depressive disorder and, thus, can only occur during a recovery.

Figure 17
The typical course of depressive disorders and the phases of treatment. (Adapted from Kupfer, 1991).

Extending the clinical use of antidepressants

It is a mistake to regard all antidepressants as the same, that is, effectively as equivalent magic bullets. The original TCAs embodied a number of therapeutic principles to the point where, if re-launched today, drugs such as imipramine, desipramine, clomipramine, trimipramine and opipramol would be classified as belonging to different groups: SNRIs, NARIs, SSRIs, noradenergic and specific serotonergic antidepressants (NASSAs) and others. The recognition of depressive disorders was poor in the 1950s, but the recognition and detection of other conditions such as obsessive–compulsive disorder, social phobia and panic disorder were even poorer. As a result, the early thymeretic (drive-enhancing) and thymoleptic (mood-seizing) agents, as they were called, became antidepressants almost by default. They were clearly different agents from the sedative anxiolytics of the barbiturate and benzodiazepine type.

Categorizing the TCAs and monoamine oxidase inhibitors (MAOIs) simply as anti-depressants was probably facilitated by the emergence of the monoamine hypotheses with their assumption of some final common biological lesion that underpinned depressive disorders. It was also facilitated by the standardization of clinical trials methodology, which took place at the end of the 1960s. Before that, the assessment of treatment effects depended primarily on clinical global impressions, which were that the antidepressants differed. In fact it was these impressions that led to the development of the SSRIs. Paul Kielholz from Basel produced a representative outline of clinical impressions in the late 1960s *(see Chapter 2) (Figure 18)*.

Arvid Carlsson, was struck by the fact that the drive-enhancing agents were active on catecholamine systems whereas those that acted on a mood component were more likely to inhibit serotonin (5HT) reuptake. It was from these observed differences that the SSRIs were developed. The initial hope was that selective 5HT agents would be more effective, act quicker and have fewer side-effects than the older, less selective agents. This is clearly not the case.

From the vantage point of the late 1990s, as mentioned in **Chapter 1**, one way to characterize the therapeutic principle embodied in the SSRIs is in terms of a broad-ranging antinervousness principle – a non-sedative anxiolytic. Other possibilities are outlined in **Chapter 7**. This broad antinervousness action has an obvious use in depressive disorders, social phobia, obsessive–compulsive disorders, panic disorders and a range of other states. The first clear proof for it came with the discovery that clomipramine was more effective in the treatment of obsessive–compulsive disorders than imipramine. Subsequent trials have indicated that desipramine is virtually ineffective in obsessive–compulsive disorders. These observations led to the use of SSRIs for obsessive–compulsive disorders. In general drugs that have actions on the serotonergic system seem to be of use in these disorders, whereas drugs selective for noradrenergic systems do not.

Initially, it was argued that the responsiveness of conditions such as obsessive–compulsive disorders to antidepressants stemmed from the fact that a depressive disorder underlay these neurotic conditions; clearing up the depression would

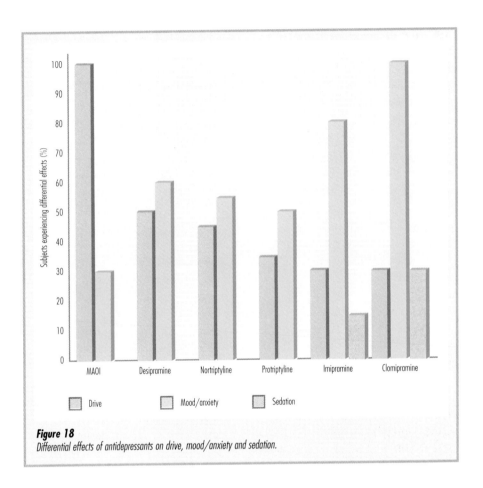

Figure 18
Differential effects of antidepressants on drive, mood/anxiety and sedation.

lead to an improvement in the neurosis. This is clearly not the case. The licences given to a number of the SSRIs for use in panic disorders, obsessive–compulsive disorders and social phobia depend on a demonstration of effectiveness after exclusion of depression.

In recent years the focus on the SSRIs has helped to clarify the nature of their effects. There has, however, been neglect of the profile of action of drugs selective for noradrenergic systems. Agents that are active on noradrenergic systems seem, in the main, to be better at enhancing vigilance, drive and motivation, a profile of action that clearly benefits people with depressive disorders *(Figure 19)*. It may also be useful in panic disorders – where, for example, lofepramine has been shown to be effective. The use of MAOIs in social phobias also supports the idea that an action on catecholamine systems could also offer distinctly useful effects in these conditions.

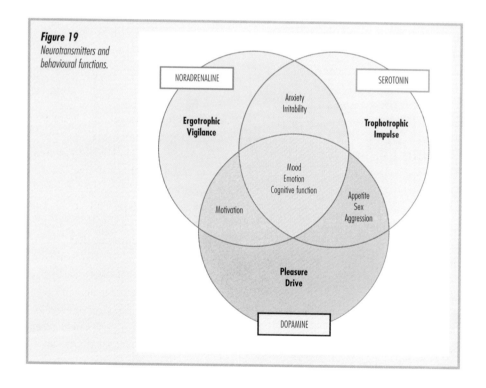

Figure 19
Neurotransmitters and behavioural functions.

Currently drugs that are selective for noradrenergic systems appear to be more beneficial in severe types of depression, as well as in those that are characterized by psychomotor retardation and obvious complaints of fatigue, in addition to a loss of interest or pleasure in normal activities – the patient who is tired all the time. It is tempting to think that greater effectiveness in melancholic or severe types of depression is the same as a greater antidepressant potency, but this is not so. Antidepressant potency is somewhat mythical. The size of treatment effect for all these agents varies with the population being studied, whether they are young or elderly people, or whether they are anergic or anxious. Some of the SSRIs have been of use in a psychotic condition called body dysmorphic disorder; this indicates that they are not 'weaker' than the TCAs or agents selective for noradrenergic systems.

Based on strong indications that agents with actions on the noradrenergic system improve depressive states characterized by fatigue or anhedonia, it could be predicted that these agents would have benefits in chronic fatigue states, in addition to their usefulness in depressive disorders. To date the SSRIs have demonstrated no such benefit. An explanation could be that some personalities are predisposed to showing signs of tiredness rather than anxiety when depressed, whereas others develop signs of anxiety.

It will be interesting to see in the future whether agents that are vigilant and drive enhancing, such as reboxetine, are of benefit to a variety of chronic fatigue syndromes as well as to conditions such as neurasthenia *(Figure 20)*. Whether there are differential effects with patients who are more typically anxious being more likely to respond to a serotonergic agent remains to be seen.

Another group of patients who deserve further investigation are those who have conditions ranging from hypochondriasis to somatization disorders. To date little work has been done in this area, although these patients and those with chronic pain syndromes use up a good deal of the time and resources of general practice. The effects of noradrenergic agents in enhancing vigilance are relevant when dealing with the external environment, but the main noradrenergic nucleus, the locus coeruleus, has more extensive inputs from the internal than from the external environment. This can be demonstrated when

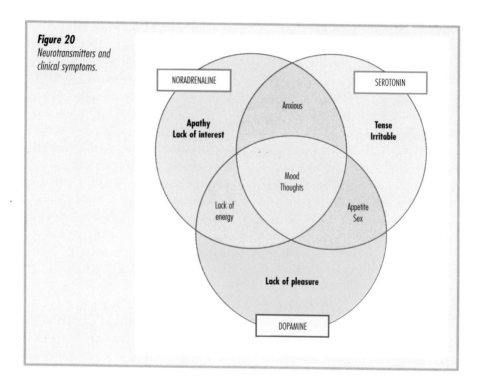

Figure 20
Neurotransmitters and clinical symptoms.

we consider how a full bladder or bowel will override our interest in a lecture on pharmacology. A possible use for noradrenergic agents could then be predicted in conditions that have prominent somatic complaints.

Personality considerations may dictate the usefulness of noradrenergic-selective agents in some conditions and of serotonergic-selective agents in others. Selective effects of this sort may help to open up the hitherto relatively neglected area of liaison psychiatry. In fact, maprotiline, a noradrenergic-selective agent, that is by far the best-selling antidepressant in Japan, sells particularly well in areas of psychosomatic medicine.

Other conditions

One way in which the action of serotonergic-active drugs can be characterized is in terms of a broad, non-sedative, antinervousness action, which underlies their use in a range of conditions. Just as morphine may have antitussive, analgesic, euphoriant and sedative effects, depending on which brain regions it acts on, so the SSRIs and noradrenergic-selective agents can also have more than one therapeutic functional effect.

The 5HT system was initially characterized as the trophotrophic or vegetative system. It is clear that the $5HT_{2C}$-receptor is centrally involved in the regulation of aspects of dysphoria, on the one hand, and appetite, on the other, whereas $5HT_{2A}$-receptors act on the slow wave components of sleep. The modulatory effects of 5HT availability as a consequence of fluoxetine use, for example, acting on $5HT_{2C}$-receptors, possibly underlies the benefit of these agents in eating disorders. Fluoxetine, in particular, has been shown to have an appetite-regulating effect which appears to be beneficial in some patients. The effects of trazodone, mianserin, mirtazapine and nefazodone on $5HT_{2A}$-receptors in practice has led to

some use of these agents to improve sleep quality, especially in the elderly.

One of the prominent effects (side-effect) of the SSRIs is their impact on sexual functioning; they are believed to produce sexual dysfunction, which involves delayed orgasm for both men and women. In a significant proportion of men, however, such effects have the potential to be therapeutically beneficial. There are estimates that up to one-third of men have premature ejaculation. Controlled trials comparing the use of clomipramine and placebo in premature ejaculation have indicated a clear use for the drug, with ejaculation being delayed significantly by use of 10–25 mg clomipramine 2–3 hours before intercourse. In a more recent trial comparing paroxetine with placebo, it was also found that the length of time to ejaculation was significantly extended in men with premature ejaculation.

In contrast antagonists at $5HT_{2A}$-receptor sites could be expected to enhance orgasm, and such agents include the antidepressants trazodone and nefazodone. They could be considered to have a mild aphrodisiac effect, in terms of increasing sexual interest in both men and women. For men with premature ejaculation this could be a problem. It could, however, be more useful for men or women who suffer loss of libido; it can also be used to manage sexual dysfunction induced by SSRIs. Buspirone, which acts as a $5HT_{1A}$-agonist, appears to have similar effects, yohimbine, which acts on $5HT_{2A}$-receptors, also has these effects.

Currently the effects of noradrenergic-selective agents on sexual functioning are not clear, and it is not known whether they have a therapeutic use.

Antidepressants have been used for a long time in chronic pain syndromes: their effectiveness has in fact led to the argument, by some investigators, that many pain syndromes are cases of masked depression. The development of the SSRIs has made it possible to explore this area more thoroughly. The relative inefficacy of the SSRIs in this area, when compared with desipramine and amitrityline, would suggest that it is the TCAs' noradrenergic component that underpinned their use in pain syndromes. These issues could possibly be clarified by further studies with reboxetine.

Noradrenergic-selective agents, such as desipramine, are used widely in the USA for hyperactivity disorders in place of

agents such as methylphenidate. This use is entirely rational if the vigilance-enhancing properties of these agents are borne in mind. Desipramine is, however, a dangerous agent in overdose and its use is therefore problematic, for children. Studies of lofepramine and reboxetine are needed.

The SSRIs have shown a greater use in the treatment of premenstrual dysphoric disorder (PMDD) than the older non-selective TCAs. Trials with selective NARIs provide an opportunity to confirm whether the selective effect of 5HT agents in PMDD arises by virtue of their general anti-irritability profile of action or because of some other action related specifically to 5HT. Alternatively it is possible that any antidepressant would work quicker in PMDD, which is brief and reactive by nature; this could be because downstream effects do not build up in these conditions as they do in chronic depressive disorders. The drawback of the older non-selective agents could have been their weight-gaining side-effects rather than any lack of effect on the condition. This point may be clarified by trials with reboxetine in PMDD.

A use of SSRIs that is not widely known is in the treatment of catalepsy. An SSRI can be used for catalepsy itself or when it is part of the narcoleptic syndrome.

The idea of noradrenergic and serotonergic types of depression has arisen from evidence that certain individuals respond better to serotonergic-selective agents and others respond to agents that act on catecholamine systems. There has been no experimental support for this idea. The work of Peter Joyce and colleagues suggests that patients with particular personality types are more likely to respond to selective noradrenergic or serotonergic agents, which may be a result of biological components of personality rather than of the depression itself. Noradrenergic personalities may be more likely to be easily tired and serotonergic personalities show greater irritability and impulsivity. Alternatively certain personality types may respond preferentially to the induction of sanguinity by serotonergic-selective agents whereas others respond better to the activating or vitality-restoring effects of noradrenergic-active agents. One way of ascertaining this is to ask patients whether the treatment suits them – does it offer them what they want from treatment?.

A general rule of thumb

To date there has been a tendency in psychiatry and primary care to assume that antidepressants get patients well by simply raising monoamine levels. No-one has asked the question: what do we want treatment to do in order to get the patient well? This is in marked contrast to the treatment of cardiac, gastrointestinal or hypertensive conditions, where physicians usually have a clear view of what they expect from the treatment – for example, reduction in acid levels or killing off *Helicobacter pylori*, for gastrointestinal conditions.

The differences emerging between drugs that select different systems are forcing clinicians to confront this functional question. This makes the decision to prescribe more reflective, but it also offers greater chances of picking the right treatment. It should be possible to involve patients in this exercise by asking them what they think needs to be done in order to get them well. Do they say 'Make me energetic and more outgoing' or 'Make me less irritable and less anxious'.

Use of antidepressants in special patient groups

Children and young adults

Psychiatric disorders, such as bipolar mood disorders, schizophrenia and obsessive–compulsive disorder, can frequently start in childhood or the early adolescent years. Commonly, however, the data sheets for anti-depressant drugs include a disclaimer against prescribing to these groups. This disclaimer should not limit medical practice in any way. The basis for prescribing for children and adolescents is the same as that employed to prescribe anticonvulsants in children who are having convulsions. When faced with such a problem no-one would hesitate to prescribe an anticonvulsant, even though, until recently, no anticonvulsant had a licence for use in childhood disorders. A drug's licence indicates the claims that a pharmaceutical manufacturer can make regarding that product, and these claims are constrained by what has been demonstrated to be the case. The freedom of a clinician to prescribe, however, stems from the Medicines Act in the UK, or its equivalent in other countries; this confers a freedom to use any agents that have been allowed on to the market place.

In the case of obsessive–compulsive disorders, there is good evidence in childhood, teenage and adult conditions that drugs with a prominent 5HT reuptake-inhibiting component may be of therapeutic benefit in this condition, whereas noradrenergic selective agents have little effect. The continuity of effects across childhood and adult conditions gives strong support to ·
the use of the SSRIs for obsessive–compulsive disorder in children and teenagers.
Likewise the use of SSRIs could be considered in exceptionally severe cases of social phobia or other anxiety disorders arising in teenagers.

However, for depressive disorders in childhood the situation is more complex. A small proportion of mood disorders in childhood present with clear stigmata of bipolarity by virtue of either a manic presentation or a cycling between depression and mania, or vice versa. In such cases there is a good argument for prescribing the full range of antidepressants that are used in adult disorders.

The larger proportion of mood disorders in children and teenagers appears to be much more reactive in nature; they respond to any pharmacological or non-pharmacological interventions. The rates of response to placebos in these age groups runs at 65%

or more, compared with 30–40% in adult populations. To date it has not been possible to demonstrate any superiority of TCAs over a placebo in these groups, but there is some evidence and an emerging consensus that the SSRIs, possibly by virtue of their more anxiolytic properties, are likely to be of greater benefit in these age groups.

Elderly people

Depressive illness in elderly people mirrors that found in childhood. In elderly people, a recourse to ECT is more likely to be needed or useful. There are also likely to be more melancholic features, in particular psychomotor retardation, and there is some evidence that agents with prominent actions on catecholaminergic systems may be of greater benefit for such populations than agents that have actions selective to the 5HT system.

Elderly people are also, however, more likely to have concurrent physical illnesses, receive concomitant medication and perhaps be at greater risk of not being diagnosed as being depressed. This may result from their mood states being seen as an inevitable consequence of other illnesses, other treatments or old age itself.

It is often important in this age group to avoid medication that carries a significant risk of cardiovascular complications – cardiac arrhythmias, orthostatic hypotension or anticholinergic-induced delirium. In many cases, therefore, an initial trial of treatment with an SSRI may be indicated, even if this needs supplementing with an agent that has effects on catecholamine systems, such as mianserin or mirtazapine. The development of agents that have selective effects, such as reboxetine, offers a significant alternative in this area.

Patients with heart disease

Depressive disorders are a common accompaniment of cardiac disorders. The association is very close and it is striking how the depressive symptomatology can predict the outcome of a cardiac problem, this means that special consideration should be given to the question of the treatment of depression when complicated by cardiac disorders. The older TCAs in general produce a tachycardia and increase the propensity to cardiac arrhythmias of one sort or the other *(see Chapter 5)*. The use of TCAs and other noradrenergic-selective agents, such as maprotiline and lofepramine, therefore

can be complicated. In contrast the SSRIs are more likely to be free of direct cardiotoxic effects and less likely to have effects on the peripheral vascular system which can cause postural hypotension. They are not, however, without their cardiovascular complications. They are more likely to lead to clotting disorders, acting through 5HT-receptors in vascular walls and platelets.

At present, there have been no studies that directly address the question of which agents are safest when the cardiovascular system is compromised. There is not a single published study demonstrating better outcomes with a particular antidepressant or even with a particular class of antidepressant. There is a case for saying that SSRIs are in general safer, but, as this group of patients is also older, they may be less effective. If the SSRIs fail, it is often necessary to consider other agents and relatively NARIs such as reboxetine, maprotiline or lofepramine are worth trying; but their use needs careful monitoring in the early stages of treatment. Moclobemide is a further option. This reversible monoamineoxidase inhibitor, unlike older MAOIs, does not cause hypotensive effects. This whole area needs to be reviewed regularly by prescribers.

Depression complicated by neurological disturbances

Depression is more common in neurological disorders than in any other disorder except for cardiac disorders. The frequency of depressive reactions after strokes, Parkinson's disease and subcortical disorders is in general extremely high. There is also a state of emotional lability, which often follows a stroke. This is not a major depressive disorder as such, but it responds to antidepressant treatments and in particular to imipramine. There is higher frequency of depressive disorders in individuals with evidence of minor brain infarcts, and the response to conventional treatments, is poorer in this kind of depression. Treatment is, however, necessary because the frequency of suicides after strokes is high.

The use of SSRIs is associated with treatment-induced dyskinesias, dystonias and akathisia. This argues against the use of SSRIs in the treatment of the depression that accompanies Parkinson's disorder and for the use of NARIs or TCAs. However, all the SSRIs do not have the same effects, fluoxetine and paroxetine being more likely, and sertraline and citalopram relatively less likely, to produce dyskinesias and akathisia *(see Chapter 5)*. In general, in depressive disorders complicated by neurological conditions, agents acting on the noradrenergic system, including MAOIs, are probably therefore a better first-line treatment. It must, however, be emphasized that this is based on theory with an absence of clear data. In subjects who are older, and have signs of early cognitive impairment, there is some evidence to suggest that citalopram may have beneficial effects that are not found with other SSRIs.

Antidepressants and suicide

Clearly, suicide is one of the hazards of a depressive episode. Before the introduction of antidepressants, it was recognized that the periods of maximum risk appeared to be the entry into and exit from depressive episodes. This led to the early speculation that antidepressants, simply by increasing the number of exits from and subsequent re-entrances into depressive episodes, might lead to an increased risk of suicide. Subsequently, it appeared that agents differed in their likelihood of triggering suicidal episodes, with the MAOIs apparently being the most likely to do so.

Of the original psychotropic agents, the first generation of antidepressants was unique in being toxic in overdose. The subsequent development of mianserin and other agents that were safer in overdose marked a step forward. Along with this progress on the issue of safety in overdose came another problem: the apparent precipitation of suicide in some individuals, not otherwise suicidal, with agents that were safe in overdose. The problem first appeared with fluoxetine in the form of a series of case reports, which linked the genesis of suicidal ideation to the development of akathisia. The evidence is as follows. Sceptics argue that there is no randomized clinical trial evidence to this effect and that the claim is based on case reports. They also argue that depressive disorders are associated with lifetime suicide prevalence rates of the order of 15% or 600 per 100 000 patient-years. Those more impressed with the possibility that any antidepressant may induce problems have noted that the case reports involved in the case of fluoxetine employed test–retest methods, that there is a consistency across the sites and that there is a plausibility to the proposed mechanism by which some antidepressants cause problems. It has been suggested, in particular, that the greatest problems may occur when treatment triggers akathisia, which is a particular hazard during the first 2 weeks of treatment. Finally, there is epidemiological evidence to support the possibility that not all antidepressants are the same. In 1995, a large survey of

primary care prescribing produced estimates that the various antidepressants were associated with suicide in the following order: lofepramine 41/100 000 patient-years; dothiepin 87/100 000 patient-years; mianserin 165/100 000 patient-years; and fluoxetine 189/100 000 patient-years. When factors such as a history of previous suicide attempts are controlled for, the figures for mianserin drop back to 95/100 000 patient-years, but those for fluoxetine remain the same. These figures received broad confirmation from a study of successful suicides in Sweden, which showed that noradrenergic-selective agents, including lofepramine and maprotiline, were associated with lower suicide rates than other agents.

The figure of 15% lifetime prevalence of suicide was taken from severely depressed patients who were hospitalized during the 1960s. Since then we have recognized the existence of milder affective disorders, a 10% annual prevalence rate for these disorders and up to a 50% lifetime prevalence rate. Based on this, and the fact that it is conventionally said that half of those who commit suicide are depressed (2500 out of 5000 in the UK), the lifetime suicide prevalence rate for all affective disorders can be estimated at about 1–1.5%. This gives an annual prevalence of 50/100 000 patient-years. Indeed, at present, the published data from community epidemiological studies do not rule out the possibility that some mild affective disorders exert a protective effect against suicide.

From these figures, there are grounds to suspect that some individuals may become suicidal on certain antidepressants. A range of drug-induced problems may be precipitating factors, from an induction of agitation (akathisia) on some SSRIs to the extremely distressing problem of urinary retention with noradrenergic-selective agents. Sexual dysfunction or depersonalization reactions may also be problematic. In all these cases, there is the implication that patients should be closely monitored, particularly during the early stages of treatment.

Certain conclusions can be drawn from the above figures:

1   Untreated moderate-to-severe depressive disorders carry a substantial risk of suicide and treatment reduces this risk. In such cases treatment efficacy should be the first determinant of choice of treatment.

2   Toxicity in overdoes is an important aspect of antidepressant treatment and should feature clearly in management decisions taken for patients who are known to be suicidal.

3   A proportion of patients may become suicidal or more suicidal on antidepressant treatment, and this may be linked to the side-effect profile of the agent being used. Management should involve an awareness of the risk, regular monitoring during the early stages of treatment and a willingness to change treatment if indicated.

4   At present noradrenergic-selective agents seem less likely to trigger suicidal responses than other agents.

Appendix

Main antidepressants and their proprietary names

	Generic name	Proprietary name
Monoamine oxidase inhibitors		
Non-selective	Phenelzine	Nardil
	Isocarboxazid	Marplan
	Nialamide	Niamide
	Pargyline	Eutonyl
	Tranylcypromine	Parnate
Selective (RIMAs)	Moclobemide	Aurorix
Tricyclic antidepressants		
	Imipramine	Tofranil
	Desipramine	Pertofran
	Clomipramine	Anafreanil
	Lofepramine	Gamanil
	Trimipramine	Surmontil
	Dothiepin	Prothiaden
	Amitriptyline	Tryptizol
	Nortriptyline	Nortrilen
	Doxepin	Sinequan
	Maprotiline	Ludiomil

	Generic name	Proprietary name
Tetracyclic antidepressants		
	Mianserin	Bolvidon, Tolvan
	Mirtazapine	Remeron, Zispin
Selective serotonin reuptake inhibitors (SSRIs)		
	Sertraline	Lustral
	Citalopram	Cipramil
	Paroxetine	Seroxat
	Fluoxetine	Prozac
	Nefazodone	Dutonin
	Fluvoxamine	Faverin
Specific noradrenaline and serotonin reuptake inhibitors (SNRIs)		
	Venlafaxine	Efexor
	Milnacipran	Ixel
Noradrenaline reuptake inhibitors (NARIs)		
	Viloxazine	Vivalan
	Reboxetine	Edronax
Atypical antidepressants		
	Trazodone	Molipaxin

Recommended reading

American Psychiatric Association. *Diagnostic and Statistical Manual of Mental Disorders*, 4th edn. APA Press, Washington, DC: 1994.

Baskys A, Remington G (eds). *Brain Mechanism and Psychotropic Drugs*. CRC Press, Boca Raton, FL, 1996.

Baumgarten HG, Goethert M (eds). *Serotoninergic Neurons and 5HT Receptors in the CNS*. Springer-Verlag, Berlin, 1997.

Bech P. Clinical effects of serotonin reuptake inhibitors. In: Dahl SG, Gram LF (eds). *Clinical Pharmacology in Psychiatry*. Springer-Verlag, Berlin,1989; pp 82–93.

Bloom FE, Kupfer DJ (eds). *Psychopharmacology: The Fourth Generation of Progress*. Raven Press, New York, 1995.

British Association of Psychopharmacology. Consensus statement on the use of psychotropic drugs for childhood disorders and learning disabilities. *J Psychopharmacol* 1997; **11**: 291–4.

British National Formulary, Number 30. British Medical Association and the Royal Pharmaceutical Society of Great Britain, London, 1995.

Carlsson A. The rise of neuropsychopharmacology: Impact on basic and clinical neuroscience. In: Healy D (ed). *The Psychopharmacologists*, Chapman & Hall, London, 1996; pp 51–80.

Cooper JR, Bloom FE, Roth RH. *The Biochemical Basis of Neuropharmacology*, 7th edn. Oxford University Press, New York, 1996.

den Boer JA, Sitsen JMA. *Handbook of Depression and Anxiety – A Biological Approach*. Marcel Dekker, New York, 1994.

Feldman RS, Meyer JS, Quenzer LF (eds). *Principles of Neuropsychopharmacology*. Sinauer Association, Sunderland, USA, 1997.

Gilman AG, Rall TW, Nies AS, Taylor P (eds). *The Pharmacological Basis of Therapeutics*, 9th edn. Pergamon Press, New York, 1996.

Healy D. *The Antidepressant Era*. Harvard University Press, Cambridge MA, 1997.

Healy D. Reboxetine, fluoxetine and social functioning as an outcome measure in antidepressant trials: implications. *Prim Care Psychiatry*, 1998; in press.

Healy D, McMonagle T. Enhancement of social functioning as a therapeutic principle in the management of depression. *Psychopharmacol* 1997; **11 (suppl 1)**: 25–31.

Jachuk SJ, Brierley H, Jachuk S, et al. The effect of hypotensive drugs on the quality of life. *J R Coll Gen Pract*, 1982; **32**: 103–5.

Joyce PR, Mulder RT, Cloninger CR. Temperament predicts clomipramine and desipramine response in major depression. *J Affect Disord*, 1994; **30**: 35–46.

Katschnig H. How useful is the concept of quality of life in psychiatry? *Curr Opin Psychiatry* 1997; **10**: 337–45.

Leonard BE. *Fundamentals of Psychopharmacology*, 2nd edn. John Wiley & Sons, Chichester, 1997.

Montgomery S, Halbreich U (eds). *Pharmacotherapy of Mood and Cognition*. American Psychiatric Press, Washington DC, 1998.

Schatzberg AF, Nemeroff CB (eds). *Textbook of Psychopharmacology*. American Psychiatric Press, Washington DC, 1995.

Stahl SM. *Essential Psychopharmacology*. Cambridge University Press, Cambridge 1996.

Stassen HH, Delini-Stula A, Angst J. Delayed onset of action of antidepressant drugs. *Eur Psychiatry* 1997; **12**: 166–76.

Westberg HGM, Den Boer JA, Murphy DL (eds). *Advances in the Neurobiology of Anxiety Disorders*. John Wiley & Sons, Chichester, 1996.

World Health Organization. *International Classification of Diseases* 10th edn. Geneva, WHO, 1993.

Index